CANCER CLINICAL TRIALS

Experimental Treatments &
How They Can Help You

CANCER CLINICAL TRIALS

Experimental Treatments & How They Can Help You

Robert Finn

O'REILLY®

Beijing • Cambridge • Farnham • Köln • Paris • Sebastopol • Taipei • Tokyo

Cancer Clinical Trials: Experimental Treatments & How They Can Help You
by Robert Finn

Copyright © 1999 Robert Finn. All rights reserved. Printed in the United States of America.

Published by O'Reilly & Associates, Inc., 101 Morris Street, Sebastopol, CA 95472.

Editor: Linda Lamb
Production Editor: Sarah Jane Shangraw
Production Services: Alicia Cech

Printing History:

September 1999:   First Edition

Library of Congress Cataloging-in-Publication Data
Finn, Robert. 1955-
    Cancer clinical trials: experimental treatments & how they can help you / Robert Finn
        p. cm.—(Patient-centered guides)
    Includes bibliographical references and index.
    ISBN 1-56592-566-1 (pbk.)
    1. Cancer—Research. 2. Cancer—Popular works. 3. Antineoplastic agents—Testing.
    4. Clinical trials.
I. Title. II. Series.
RC267.F56 1999
616.99'406—dc21

                                  99-38927
                                   CIP

*Dedicated to everyone who has ever
participated in a cancer clinical trial.
You are all heroes.*

Table of Contents

Foreword

IT IS A FIGURE CITED ROUTINELY nowadays at meetings of cancer advocates, physicians, and drug company executives. Only 3 percent of adult cancer patients in the United States take part in clinical trials, even though every one of those groups professes to want the number to be much higher. In the face of cancer survival statistics far below what anyone would want, why do we have such minimal enrollment in clinical trials? How will we ever know what works, goes the argument, if we are not trying new treatments?

In fact, powerful forces in American medicine often impede the progress of clinical trials and increase the difficulty at every step. Few realize that the entire concept of basing medicine on the scientific rigor of clinical trials is a recent phenomenon—beginning after the Second World War. Until then the backbone of clinical practice was that the physician knows what is best for the patient—no matter how he or she happened to gain that knowledge. Entering a patient into a clinical trial is first and foremost the admission by a physician of at least partial ignorance and a willingness to try to overcome it.

More recently, negative financial considerations helped provoke many physicians' reluctance. This is especially so in the specialty of cancer treatment, or oncology. As the practice of oncology grew and specialists moved out of academic medical centers into the community, doctors willing to suggest clinical trials for their patients often lost income and control of the patient's care. To try to overcome this difficulty, drug companies and their intermediaries, contract research organizations, often paid community doctors to enroll patients. The payments cover the additional time and effort required to collect massive amounts of information from each experimental patient, as opposed to standard records for routine treatment. Occasionally, however, the payments exceed the actual costs and include inducements to enroll trial participants. Some doctors even receive invitations to meetings in sunny resorts with expenses paid for them and a companion. These additional payments have led to inevitable allegations that they lead to biased results.

Drug companies, of course, are eager to complete clinical trials. They offer the only source of raw data that can lead to Food and Drug Administration approval of a drug and possible billions of dollars in profits. But before the companies embark on a trial, they must convince themselves that it is worth the gamble—upwards of a $200 million gamble. For smaller biotechnology companies, one trial can make the difference between survival and failure. Companies want to test just enough to win FDA approval. They have no interest in paying the enormous expense of testing their drug on more subjects than the minimum needed for FDA approval. Despite much talk of compassionate access to drugs before they win approval, such programs for cancer drugs occur very seldom—almost never. So a cancer patient seeking to get a drug being tested in a clinical trial may find a very narrow window of opportunity slammed shut.

From the patient's perspective, no matter what anyone says, all trials are not necessarily beneficial. Large academic medical centers carry out phase I, the initial testing of cancer drugs, on patients who are usually close to death. The idea is to find out whether the drug is even more toxic than the cancer. Anecdotes exist about patients in phase I who experience spectacular results, but they are rare. Numerous studies show that while volunteers for phase I are clearly told in writing and in person that they can expect no benefit from their participation, they participate because they cling to the hope that it is their last chance at survival. Even in later phase trials, the advantages to the patient may not be as clear as the patient would want. Some trials compare doses of combinations of drugs already on the market. While the results may benefit medicine as a whole, they could do little for the individual participants.

In this excellent book, Robert Finn offers an indispensable guide for the cancer patient who must negotiate these and the many other potential quagmires in first finding and then taking part in a clinical trial. I highly recommend this book as a first step in what will be for many a difficult, but crucially important, part of their struggle to beat their cancer. For despite all the obstacles, both individual patients and the medical establishment need clinical trials. They represent our only hope of overcoming the many aspects of the dreaded set of diseases we call cancer.

—Robert Bazell
Chief Science Correspondent for NBC News
Author of *Her-2: The Making of Herceptin, a Revolutionary Treatment for Breast Cancer* (Random House, 1998)

Preface

THIS BOOK IS INTENDED for anyone with a diagnosis of cancer or anyone helping such a person make medical decisions. Sometimes, the person with cancer is too wrapped up in pain, worry, and fear to be able to focus clearly on his or her medical options. It falls then to a family member or trusted friend, working in cooperation with medical professionals, to identify the decisions to be made and to present them clearly to the patient.

This book is not a guide to individual clinical trials. You won't be getting highly specific advice like, "If you have cancer X, you should be participating in trial Y," or "Forget about clinical trials on agent ZZ1234 because it doesn't work." There are many different kinds of cancer, and at any one time, there are about 1,500 different cancer clinical trials being conducted in the United States. Because new potential treatments are continually being developed, and older ones are either being approved for use or discarded, the clinical trials available to people with cancer will continually change. A guide to specific clinical trials would be out of date even before it could be published.

Nor does this book contain a case study of any one clinical trial. For an intimate look at the development of a single cancer therapy, read an outstanding book on Herceptin by NBC science correspondent Robert Bazell entitled *Her-2: The Making of Herceptin, a Revolutionary Treatment for Breast Cancer* (Random House, 1998).

Instead, this book will give you the tools you need to find and evaluate clinical trials for your particular type of cancer any time you need that information.

This book is organized so that you may read it either straight through or go directly to the chapter that contains subjects of interest.

Chapter 1, *Overview of Clinical Trials*, discusses cancer clinical trials in general terms, explains why too few people participate in clinical trials, and argues that anyone with cancer should at least consider clinical trials along with other treatment options.

Chapter 2, *The Structure of Clinical Trials*, introduces you to the three main phases of clinical trials. It describes how they're conducted and the advantages and disadvantages of each phase. You'll also learn about placebos, randomization, and blinded and open-label trials.

Chapter 3, *Clinical Trial Ethics*, shows you how the current clinical trial system evolved and how the ethical codes for clinical trials developed. You'll learn about the rights and responsibilities of all the parties involved in clinical trials and where to complain if something goes wrong.

Chapter 4, *How to Find Clinical Trials*, shows you numerous ways of identifying clinical trials that might be useful for your medical condition.

Chapter 5, *Special Types of Trials*, describes the unique considerations involved in specialized types of clinical trials, including genetic trials, prevention trials, and trials of new diagnostic devices.

Chapter 6, *Choosing Possible Trials*, discusses general considerations in choosing a clinical trial and the special considerations involved in clinical trials for children and for people with advanced cancer.

Chapter 7, *Evaluating a Clinical Trial*, shows you how to make a decision about whether to participate in a specific clinical trial. You'll find a thorough dissection of an informed consent form, and you'll learn how to make sense of trials' highly technical protocol documents. This chapter also includes a long list of questions to ask the people running the trial, and concludes with a list of questions to ask yourself to help make the decision whether to participate.

Chapter 8, *Administration of Clinical Trials*, shows you how clinical trials are organized, managed, and regulated.

Chapter 9, *Financial Issues*, describes the economic considerations involved in clinical trial participation. Among other things, you'll learn how to find out if your insurance will cover clinical trials, and you'll learn some strategies for dealing with the situation if it doesn't.

Appendix A, *Resources*, collects in a single location an annotated list of resources related to clinical trials.

Appendix B, *Critical Public Documents*, presents the actual text of some of the most important documents regulating the conduct of clinical trials.

Acknowledgments

This book owes a great deal to a great many people. First and foremost, I'd like to thank Linda Lamb, editor of the Patient-Centered Guides series. In twenty years as a science and medical writer, I've had the good fortune of working with some fine editors, but Linda has been the best of all. From our initial discussions through the final revisions, Linda's ideas have improved this book immeasurably. Her friendliness and good nature were instrumental in making this project a delight from beginning to end.

I'd also like to thank everyone else at O'Reilly & Associates, especially Carol Wenmoth and Lisa Olson, who worked so hard to get this book to its readers.

A large number of people with a wide variety of experiences related to cancer clinical trials proved willing to spend time answering my questions, telling their stories, reviewing sections of the manuscript, and providing various other forms of assistance, small and large. In particular, I'd like to thank Jane H. Bick, PhD; Dina Butin; Gregory T. David; Donald Drake; Steve Dunn; Sharon K. Friend; Richard A. Gams, MD; Ken Getz; Pam Geyer; Beth Gonda; Maria A. Infantine-Harwood; David Jablons, MD; Robert M. Johnson; Robert L. Kuhn; Vita J. Land, MD; Alice LaRocca; Joyce R. Niblack; Michael S. Noel; Nancy Oster; Ephraim Resnik, MD; Lydia Cunningham Rising; Victor M. Santana, MD; Gary Schine; Dale Shoemaker, PhD; Abigail A. Silvers, MD; Abby Sinnott; Paul Sonnenschein; Don Sterner; Janet Twombly; Harold Y. Vanderpool, PhD, ThM; Kesinee Yip; and Harry Youtt. Several other people provided valuable assistance but for various reasons have asked not to be mentioned by name. I thank them as well.

I also owe a debt of gratitude to the many people who shared their experiences in the lively CANCER-L mailing list and in the Usenet newsgroups alt.support.cancer and sci.med.diseases.cancer. I have learned an enormous amount by lurking in those forums.

Despite the contributions of so many people, any errors that remain are my own.

Finally, I'd like to thank Joanne Cosmos Finn, my darling wife, whose love and support are a constant source of inspiration, and without whom this book would certainly not have been written.

CHAPTER ONE

Overview of Clinical Trials

IF YOU OR A FAMILY MEMBER has been diagnosed with cancer, you probably have many questions and want to make sure you are making the best possible decisions for treatment. This book is aimed at helping you consider the range of treatment options available through clinical trials—treatments that might not be available any other way.

This chapter first describes clinical trials in general terms. After looking at reasons people don't participate in trials, it includes the reasons why you should at least consider available clinical trials as part of your decision making about cancer treatments. The chapter closes with a short discussion of traditional and alternative, or complementary, medicine.

Real promise in new treatments

Although cancer continues to be a frightening disease, cancer research now offers genuine hope for better cures. Basic research on cell biology is finally yielding important clues about the nature of cancer, and these clues are leading directly to promising new treatments. Physicians are finding better ways to alleviate cancer pain and some of the toxic side effects of chemotherapy. Medical device companies are testing new ways to detect cancer in ever earlier stages. And researchers are even creating therapies that will prevent the development of cancer in people who are at risk.

None of these new developments leaps from the scientist's mind to the clinic in a single step. The brightest of bright ideas must be tested in the laboratory, first in the test tube and then on animal models of cancer. Only if these preliminary tests give some evidence that the new treatment works and is reasonably safe is it tried on human beings—in a clinical trial.

Current statistics

Clinical trials of new therapies—and the hope they bring—are important because cancer statistics are stark and unpleasant. According to the American Cancer Society (ACS) and the National Cancer Institute (NCI), cancer is the second leading cause of death in the United States, exceeded only by heart disease. In 1998, there were an estimated 564,800 deaths from cancer, fully one quarter of all the deaths in the US. More than 1.2 million Americans were newly diagnosed with cancer in 1998, and a total of 8 million living Americans have a history of cancer.

In the 1930s, only 25 percent of cancer patients survived five years. The five-year survival rate rose to 40 percent in the 1990s, but much of that modest improvement may be due not to better treatment, but to the fact that we're able to detect cancer much earlier these days. Earlier detection means a longer period of survival after diagnosis, even if the course of the disease remains exactly the same.

Despite decades of intensive research, despite the War on Cancer declared by President Richard Nixon in 1971, and despite generous funding, dedicated investigators, and courageous patients, improvements in cancer treatment have been only incremental, and cures remain elusive. One thing is certain, however: every potential new therapy must pass the rigorous test of clinical trials before it can come into wide usage.

What is a clinical trial?

New treatments aren't tried casually or haphazardly. Legitimate researchers don't say, "I'm really excited about my laboratory results with Compound X. Joe Smith here has cancer. Let's see if it'll cure him!" Hundreds of years of experience with the scientific method have taught researchers that to learn something about the physical world, you have to ask precise, narrow questions. You have to design an experiment that will give you an unambiguous answer to those questions, and then you have to run that experiment carefully so it genuinely answers the questions you're asking. When the subjects of the experiments are human beings, you must also take into account important practical and ethical considerations.

Experiments that are conducted on human beings, and that are intended to answer a therapeutic question, are called clinical trials. Essentially, investigators must answer three types of questions, in order, in clinical trials:

1. Is the new treatment safe?

2. Is the new treatment effective?

3. Is the new treatment better than other treatments?

New treatments reach the general public only if all three of the questions can be answered affirmatively.

If all human beings were the same, you could get away with conducting those experiments on just a handful of people, and you'd have your answer in short order. Give Mary a dose of Compound X. If she doesn't get sick, it's safe. Give Alice several doses. If her cancer goes away, it's effective. Give Sam Compound X and give Jim the current standard treatment. If Sam does better than Jim, Compound X is better than the standard treatment.

Unfortunately, human beings are complex biological organisms, and cancer is a puzzling and often perverse disease. A certain drug might make some people very sick, while others tolerate it well. Cancers sometimes go away spontaneously, even without any treatment at all. Drugs that work extremely well in destroying one person's cancer might have no effect on another person.

The only way to get reliable answers to the questions that are asked in clinical trials is to try the new treatment on hundreds or thousands of people. If most people don't get sick, it's safe. If it makes most people's cancer go away, it's effective. If on average people do better with Compound X than with the standard treatment, then Compound X is better. This is an extremely expensive and lengthy process that costs hundreds of millions of dollars and can take many years. According to the Pharmaceutical Research and Manufacturers of America (PhRMA), it takes an average of fifteen years to bring an experimental drug out of the lab.

Why do clinical trials take so long?

Everyone wishes drug approvals could move along much more swiftly. If they did, ineffective treatments could be discarded and effective treatments would reach people with cancer sooner.

Some of the factors that retard progress are administrative. As described in Chapter 8, *Administration of Clinical Trials*, the US Food and Drug Administration (FDA) has developed a complex, lengthy, and expensive process that pharmaceutical companies must follow before new drugs are approved for sale. Although this process is intended to keep unsafe and ineffective drugs off the market, many activists charge that the FDA's regulations have the effect of keeping lifesaving treatments away from the people who need them most.

In response to these criticisms, in 1996 the FDA made it easier to demonstrate a new treatment's effectiveness. Before the new rules went into effect, pharmaceutical companies had to demonstrate an actual increase in survival time for a cancer treatment to be considered effective. The new rules allow researchers to use "surrogate markers"—such as tumor shrinkage—as a somewhat more indirect indication of effectiveness. This is expected to speed up the drug approval process significantly.

The FDA's rules are not the only reason that it takes so long to evaluate a potential cancer treatment. According to the NCI, fewer than 5 percent of adult cancer patients ever participate in a clinical trial.[1] According to some estimates, if just twice the number of cancer patients could be persuaded to participate, new treatments could be evaluated in half the time it takes now.

Many factors hold down the number of clinical trial participants, and it's unclear which are the most significant. Among them, in no particular order, are:

- **Lack of awareness**. Some cancer patients might not be aware that clinical trials are an option.

- **Reluctance to second-guess the physician**. Some cancer patients might fear that asking their physicians about clinical trials would be perceived as a criticism of the treatment they're receiving.

- **Unreceptive physicians**. Some physicians—amazingly, even some oncologists—express distaste for clinical trials. As cancer survivor Gary Schine recalls, "When I mentioned clinical trials, my doctor told me, 'I don't want my patients being treated like guinea pigs.'" (Schine's story is told in more detail in Chapter 4, *How to Find Clinical Trials*.)

- **Reluctance to refer**. Some physicians might be hesitant to refer their patients to clinical trials at other institutions. Even when they are willing to suggest a clinical trial, they might only suggest trials in which they are personally involved.

- **Overly strict eligibility requirements**. Some clinical trial protocols allow investigators to enroll only patients with specific medical histories. As described in Chapter 7, *Evaluating a Clinical Trial*, some critics of the current system believe that there are good reasons to broaden inclusion and exclusion criteria, allowing more patients to participate.

- **Difficulty finding clinical trials**. Many patients—and some-times even their physicians—don't know where to go to find lists of clinical trials for which they're eligible. Fortunately, as described in Chapter 4, the search is much simpler now than it used to be. A toll-free phone call to the NCI's Cancer Information Service or a check of sites on the Internet can yield good lists of clinical trials targeted to your condition.

- **No clinical trials available**. For some types of cancer, or for some people with certain medical histories, there may be no clinical trials currently being conducted. New trials are announced continually, however, and if you want to participate in a clinical trial, it's worthwhile repeating your search on a weekly or monthly basis.

- **Distance from major medical centers**. Many patients don't live near major academic medical centers, where most clinical trials are conducted. In response, the NCI developed the Community Clinical Oncology Program (CCOP) that can often allow an oncologist far from a major medical center to administer experimental treatments locally. But some oncologists aren't hooked into CCOP, and some trials can be conducted only at certain central locations, necessitating difficult and expensive travel.

- **Difficulty with insurance coverage**. Many insurance compa-nies and health maintenance organizations (HMOs) refuse to pay for experimental treatments or even for routine care when experimental medications are free. See Chapter 9, *Financial Issues*, for strategies and tactics for dealing with problems with your insurance coverage.

- **Other financial burdens**. Some trials might involve extra clinic visits, and these can result in lost wages or child care costs.

- **Poor explanation of disease or prognosis**. If you're not given honest information about how serious your disease is and how effective or ineffective current standard treatments are, you might be unlikely to consider clinical trials.

- **A good prognosis**. If you have a type of cancer that is almost always cured by the standard treatment, there is little reason for you to consider a clinical trial.

- **A desire to stop fighting**. Some people with cancer make a rational decision to stop treatments and to accept disease progression. There are, however, some clinical trials—such as those of new treatments for cancer pain—that might be appropriate even if you have made that choice.

- **Reluctance to be randomized or to receive a placebo**. Many people fear that if they enroll in a clinical trial, they might be assigned randomly to receive less effective or inactive medication. As discussed in Chapter 2, *The Structure of Clinical Trials*, this fear is often misplaced.

- **Fear of side effects**. New treatments have unknown side effects, and learning about these is one of the main aims of clinical trials. But as Gary Schine likes to point out, "In this country, far more people have been helped than hurt by clinical trials."

Should you consider a clinical trial?

There might be many reasons not to participate in clinical trials, but there are also plenty of reasons to seek them out. You will have the opportunity to get a new treatment years before it's available to the general public. Although it won't be a clearly proven treatment, it will be one that knowledgeable physicians regard as promising. While you're in the clinical trial, you'll most likely benefit from an especially high level of medical care. And even if the treatment does not help you personally, you can take comfort in the fact that your participation will help other people with cancer down the road. Medical science cannot advance without the altruism of clinical trial participants.

Please note that we do not urge everyone with cancer to participate in clinical trials. Many of the reasons not to participate are valid, and the decision to participate in a clinical trial is a personal one. If you have cancer, you must make that decision yourself, in consultation with friends, relatives, physicians, and spiritual advisors. It's a decision that depends on many factors, which are thoroughly explored throughout this book.

It is the opinion of many medical professionals that if you have cancer, you should at least consider the available clinical trials, along with all your other treatment options. If you are not evaluating potential experimental treatments alongside the standard treatment protocols, you're simply making a decision without access to all the facts.

Some physicians, such as Dr. David Jablons, a thoracic surgeon at the University of California, San Francisco, express an even stronger point of view:

> I think that all patients with cancer should be in a clinical trial.
> If they're not in a clinical trial, it implies that we know how to
> treat the disease, which for all but a few cancers, we don't.

Thankfully, there are a few cancers for which the standard treatments are highly successful. For example, caught early, many skin cancers can be removed completely before they spread. This illustrates how critical it is to get honest information about your prognosis—a forecast of the course of your disease and an estimate of your chance for recovery—from your doctor. Lydia Cunningham Rising, a patient advocate, observes:

> The worse your prognosis is, the more you should consider a
> clinical trial. But some doctors don't like to quote statistics. I
> understand they don't want to make the patient feel like a statistic,
> but if you do not know that you have a cancer with a 2 percent
> five-year survival rate, you aren't really going to think about
> clinical trials. When that is hidden, doctors are taking away the
> patient's ability to decide what to do.

If you can't get a straight answer from your doctor, a book sponsored by the American Cancer Society, *Informed Decisions: The Complete Book of Cancer Diagnosis, Treatment, and Recovery* (Viking Penguin Books, 1997), written by Gerald P. Murphy, MD, Lois B. Morris, and Dianne Lange, is an excellent source of information on specific cancers, their standard treatments, and their likely outcomes. It's available in many libraries and bookstores.

Although a poor prognosis increases the chance that you'll want to consider clinical trials, it doesn't necessarily follow that you should ignore this option if your prognosis is good. There are clinical trials of adjuvant therapies that are focused on preventing recurrence of disease. There are prevention studies. There are studies focused on alleviating the side effects of other therapies. Clinical trials are not end-of-life options only, and anyone with a diagnosis of cancer should at least consider clinical trials.

Traditional and alternative medicine

Many doctors have a strong bias in favor of what is typically called traditional or conventional medicine. Those adjectives are misnomers, however. Modern medicine is anything but traditional or conventional.

Modern medicine depends on the scientific method, which is certainly one of the crowning glories of human thought. The scientific method gives us an extremely efficient way of asking precise questions about how nature works, and wielded correctly, it yields precise answers. Using the scientific method, modern medicine has rapidly made great strides in treating individual illnesses and improving general human welfare.

In fact, it is alternative medicine that tends to be far more tradition-bound. Many advocates of alternative medicine point proudly to the fact that their chosen methodologies have been practiced for hundreds or thousands of years and contain the wisdom of the ancients. Now, *that's* traditional. Of course, the ancients believed that many physical illnesses could be treated by draining people of their excess blood. And they believed that people who were mentally ill should have holes cut into their skulls to let the demons escape. Clearly, some of the ancients weren't all that wise.

That is certainly not to say that all alternative medicine is worthless. On the contrary, many of modern medicine's greatest successes rest on traditional foundations. The ancient Greeks used a form of aspirin contained in willow bark to alleviate pain. Digitalis, which increases the contraction of the heart in congestive heart failure, is derived from the foxglove plant and was used by generations of women healers in England. Curare, an important drug used for muscle relaxation during anesthesia, was discovered by studying the poisoned arrows of South American hunters. There's an entire branch of science called ethnopharmacology, whose goal is to study traditional remedies in search of new medicines for modern-day ailments.

This is also not to suggest that people with cancer should avoid alternative medicine. First of all, there are clinical trials of various alternative medicines underway, and people should consider participating in them. It's only through such clinical trials that the alternatives can be proven safe and effective—and incorporated into the mainstream—or proven unsafe or ineffective and discarded.

Secondly, even alternative methods that are unproven might have beneficial effects. For example, there may not be any studies proving that quiet meditation is an effective cancer treatment. However, meditation is soothing and relaxing, and a person with cancer might be very well served by investigating various meditation techniques. Alternative medicine may also be a way of harnessing the mysterious placebo effect (discussed in more detail in Chapter 2, *The Structure of Clinical Trials*).

Rather than relying solely on alternative medicine, however, it makes more sense to use it in combination with modern medicine.

This is referred to as complementary medicine. Michael Lerner's excellent book, *Choices in Healing: Integrating the Best of Conventional and Complementary Approaches to Cancer* (MIT Press, 1994) gives a thorough overview of integrating conventional and complementary approaches to cancer treatments. It's available in many libraries and bookstores, as well as online, in its entirety, at *http://www.commonweal.org/choicescontents.html*.

If you do choose to rely in part on complementary medicine, it's critical that you tell your doctor about it. Some "herbal" remedies, for example, contain powerful chemicals that might conflict with your other treatments. Just because something is derived from an herb or is freely available in a health-food store, it doesn't mean that it's safe.

Finally, it's a sad fact that although many alternative medicine practitioners are well-intentioned, others are despicable snake-oil salesmen who cynically exploit the credulity and desperation of people with cancer. Unfortunately, in the absence of data from valid clinical trials, it's difficult to separate the good from the bad in alternative medicine.

If you do choose to investigate clinical trials, be sure to look carefully at the credentials of the investigators and the reputations of the sponsoring institutions.

CHAPTER TWO

The Structure of Clinical Trials

TO DETERMINE WHETHER a newly developed cancer treatment is any good, scientists must put it through a highly formalized series of experiments with human cancer patients. Only if a potential new treatment is proved to be safe, effective, and better than current treatments will it be released to the public. This chapter describes the typical sequence of events involved in taking a new treatment from the laboratory to general use. When cancer patients participate in clinical trials, they generally participate in the kinds of trials described in this chapter.

However, some clinical trials are different. These include trials of new medical devices, trials for the early detection of cancer, trials of methods for screening the population at large for certain types of cancer, and trials of treatments that might help prevent cancer. These are described further in Chapter 5, *Special Types of Trials*.

Clinical trial phases

The pathway of a potential cancer treatment from the laboratory to the clinic is typically a long and torturous one. One common misconception about clinical trials is that they are shot-in-the-dark experiments on unknown substances. On the contrary, before a new treatment is tried on people it has typically survived years of testing in the laboratory and on animals. Only the most promising of these treatments is ever tried on human beings. Of 5,000 substances tested in animals, only 5 are approved for Phase I clinical trials.

Once testing on people begins, Phase I trials first must assess the safety of the new treatment. Of 100 potential new treatments, 70 pass Phase I testing.

Then, Phase II trials must show the treatment to be effective. Only 33 of the 70 treatments that enter phase II are sufficiently effective to pass to the next stage.

Even an effective treatment will never come into common use unless Phase III trials show it to be better than the treatments that are already out there. A treatment might be judged to be better if more patients respond to it, or if they respond for a longer period of time, or if the new treatment is less toxic and has fewer side effects than the old one. Only 25 of those 33 treatments successfully pass phase III. Another way of putting it is that three out of four experimental cancer treatments are found to be unsafe, ineffective, or no better than current treatments.

Finally, Phase IV trials keep track of the treatment once the US Food and Drug Administration allows it to be used in the population at large.

Placebos: Misplaced worries

Placebo is a Latin word that means "I shall please." For thousands of years, people have gone to doctors and demanded medication even when they're not sick or when there is no medicine that can cure them. To please these patients, doctors would give them simple sugar pills, and their unknowing patients would leave satisfied.

You might be reluctant to consider clinical trials for fear that you may be given a placebo instead of active medication. But this fear is misplaced. People with cancer are unlikely to find themselves in placebo-controlled clinical trials.

You may have learned that for any scientific experiment to be valid, an experimental group must be compared to a control group. As you will see, this is not always the case in cancer clinical trials, but it's useful to understand the concept of controlled experiments just the same. To illustrate how a controlled experiment works with a simple example, suppose you wanted to figure out how well a new headache medication worked. You couldn't just give a single group of people a couple of the new pills and ask them whether their heads still hurt. First of all, there's the possibility that simply taking a pill could cause psychological effects that would relieve headache pain. Second, because there are already several good headache medications out there, you'd want to prove that the new pill works better than the old ones.

For the experiment to have scientific validity, you have to make two kinds of comparisons. First, you could compare people who took the new pill with people who took a phony pill. Something similar is done in many types of clinical trials: researchers compare a new medication to an inactive one, a placebo. If the people who took the headache pill had less severe headaches on average than the ones who took the placebo, you would have proven that the new medication had more than just a psychological effect. Experiments of this type are called "placebo controlled."

Placebos are necessary in many kinds of clinical trials because—for hotly debated reasons—doctors find that people receiving inactive medications often experience improvement in their conditions.[1] This is known as the placebo effect, and the classic paper on this phenomenon concluded that approximately 30 to 35 percent of the population respond to placebos, at least temporarily.[2] For an experimental treatment to be declared effective after a placebo-controlled clinical trial, the individuals receiving the active treatment must show significantly better results on average than those receiving the placebo.

To return to the example, to prove that the new medication was better at relieving headaches than aspirin, acetaminophen (Tylenol), or ibuprofen (Motrin), you'd have one group of people take the new medication, and you'd have several other groups take the established medications. Something similar is done in many kinds of clinical trials: researchers compare a new treatment to the standard treatments. If those taking the new medication had, on average, less severe headaches than those taking the established medications, and the difference between the groups was found to be statistically significant, then you might be able to say that the new pill was the best headache medication. Experiments of this type are said to have "active controls."

There are several reasons why it's unusual to find a placebo-controlled cancer trial. For one thing, Phase I and Phase II cancer trials hardly ever use any type of control, and typically, all the participants in those trials receive the active treatment. (See the detailed discussions of clinical trial phases later in this chapter.) Even in Phase III cancer trials, placebos are rarely used. One reason is that cancer treatments tend to have so many side effects that anyone receiving the placebo would figure it out in short order. A more important reason is that it would be unethical to deprive any person with such a serious illness of the best available treatment.

Instead, Phase III clinical trials for cancer typically compare the experimental treatment under study with the best available standard treatment. This is called an active-control clinical trial because even people assigned to the control group receive active treatment.

There are several exceptions to the rule that cancer clinical trials do not use placebos. Placebos might be used in trials involving those rare cancers for which no treatments are known to have any effect whatsoever, for which the best available treatment is no treatment. Fortunately, that's the case in a steadily diminishing percentage of cancers. In addition, placebos might be used in cancer prevention trials in which the participants are healthy to begin with.

Randomization

Whenever a clinical trial has an active control or a placebo control, a patient has no choice about which group—which "arm" of the study—she's assigned to. Neither does her doctor, the primary investigator, nor the pharmaceutical company sponsoring the study. Instead, a computer randomly assigns patients to one arm of the study or another. This is another way of preventing bias from creeping in. If any individual had the responsibility of assigning patients to one arm or another, he might, for example, subconsciously assign the healthier patients to the experimental arm, and at the end of the study, the experimental treatment might seem more effective than it really was.

The fear of randomization is one of the most significant factors preventing cancer patients from considering clinical trials.[3] Physicians also cite reluctance to permit randomization as a major reason they fail to refer their patients to clinical trials.[4] If you're concerned about randomization, you should consider the following points:

- Randomization is typically an issue only in Phase III trials. Phase I trials are never randomized, and Phase II trials are almost never randomized.

- Phase III trials are randomized because the investigators don't know whether the experimental treatment is better than the standard treatment. If the experimental treatment were known to be better, there'd be no need for a clinical trial.

- Anyone considering a clinical trial should examine the informed consent and protocol documents carefully for detailed information about randomization. For example, if a particular trial were designed to compare an experimental treatment with two different standard treatments, you might have only a one-third chance of receiving the experimental treatment.

- Phase III is the first time the experimental treatment is given to large numbers of patients. There may well be serious side effects to the experimental treatment that had not shown up previously.

- If one treatment proves to be significantly superior to the others during the course of the study, the Data Safety and Monitoring Board will terminate the trial early, and all patients will have the opportunity to receive the superior treatment.

Steve Dunn, a cancer survivor who maintains *CancerGuide*, a cancer information web site (*http://cancerguide.org/*), says it's important to remember that anyone has the freedom to leave a clinical trial at any time. This freedom suggests the following strategy to avoid being randomized into the less desirable arm of a clinical trial:

> You would have to decide if your conscience permits you to do this, but you could enter the trial and then quit if you didn't get what you wanted. But even if you think it would be ethical, you should only consider doing this if you knew for sure that you had some better option. I think it's dishonest, but that doesn't mean it's wrong.

You shouldn't expect, however, to be able to go from center to center in a multicenter trial, rolling the dice until you end up in the "right" treatment arm. Even if the trial organizers didn't realize what was happening, your insurance company would be unlikely to tolerate this. (See Chapter 3, *Clinical Trial Ethics*, regarding the ethics of this practice.)

Blinded and open-label trials

In clinical trials that compare two or more treatments or compare an active medication to a placebo, there is always a danger that too much knowledge might bias the results. People who know they're receiving the experimental treatment might be more hopeful, whereas people who know they're receiving the standard treatment might have a greater tendency to become discouraged. That difference in mental attitude alone might cause the patients in the first group to do better than those in the second.

For that reason, the patients participating in some clinical trials are not told which treatment group they are in. In clinical-trial lingo, this is called blinding. When only the patients are kept in the dark about which treatment they're receiving, the study is referred to as a single-blind trial.

Patients in a clinical trial are often not the only ones who are kept in the dark. The investigators and the clinical staff might try to maintain scientific detachment, but they're human, and they too hope that the experimental treatment they're testing will be an improvement over the standard treatment. Bias can creep in if they communicate their hopes to the patients. With a wink or a nod, a nurse or a technician might let a patient know which treatment group he's in. Even if staff members try mightily to keep the secret, they might unconsciously treat patients in the different groups differently, perhaps presenting a cheerier face to patients receiving the experimental treatment.

An investigator's bias might also appear when he records or interprets clinical data. Is that patient flushed, or does she have a naturally ruddy complexion? If the research nurse knows that the standard treatment tends to give patients a slight fever, perhaps he'll be more likely to note skin flushing for a patient in the standard group. For these reasons, the investigators are also sometimes kept in the dark about which patients are receiving which treatments. When both the patients and the clinical staff are blinded, the study is referred to as a double-blind trial.

How is it possible to keep the clinical staff—and the patients—in the dark about treatments? It's relatively simple if both the experimental and standard treatments involve simple medications that are administered at regular times during the day. Someone who's not directly involved in the care of patients in the study will prepare the medications, and they'll be designed to look alike. Additionally, instead of putting the names of the medications on the labels, she'll use a code. Neither the patients nor the clinical staff will know which medications they're receiving until the code is broken at the end of the study.

If the various experimental regimens being compared are complex and very different from one another—as in many cancer trials—or if they have very different side effects, keeping the patients and the clinical staff blinded will be difficult or impossible. For example, suppose the study is comparing chemotherapy alone with chemotherapy plus radiation. It will be obvious to everyone which group each patient is in. For that reason, single-blind and double-blind studies are relatively rare in cancer clinical trials. Clinical trials that are not blinded are known as open-label trials.

Investigators might use blinding if they were conducting a trial of an antinausea medication, where knowing that you got something rather than nothing might make a psychological difference. But when they're trying to measure what happens to your tumor, there's little need to be blind.

Phase I

The most important thing to know about Phase I trials is that they are not intended to demonstrate whether the treatment works. They are primarily intended to see how toxic the treatment is. Investigators use Phase I clinical trials to determine the maximally tolerated dose of a compound (MTD) and its major side effects, and to test the best means of administering the treatment (intravenously, by pills, etc.). If a patient's cancer goes into remission as the result of a Phase I clinical trial, everyone will be delighted, but that is not the main point of the study.

Although all Phase I trials concentrate on toxicity rather than efficacy, there's an important difference between Phase I cancer trials and trials for less serious conditions. For less serious conditions, the participants in the clinical trial are typically healthy volunteers, and it's not until Phase II that the treatment is given to people with the condition the treatment is intended for.

Because most potential cancer treatments by their nature are highly toxic, it would be unethical to test them on healthy subjects. For that reason, investigators typically recruit people with advanced cancer to participate in Phase I cancer trials.

What kind of person would be eligible for a Phase I cancer trial? Most likely, it would be a patient who has exhausted all known beneficial therapy or someone with a cancer for which there is no known beneficial therapy. But you wouldn't necessarily have to be terminal with a life expectancy of only a certain number of weeks.

Phase I trials typically include a relatively small number of patients, usually no more than 10 to 30. From animal experiments, the investigators will have developed an estimate of the proper dose for humans. The patients will generally be divided into several groups. The first group will receive a relatively low dose of the treatment. If it shows no unacceptable side effects, the second group will be given a higher dose, and so on. This dose escalation continues until one group shows an unacceptable level of side effects. The dose used in the previous group is then designated the MTD.

Steve Dunn began investigating cancer treatments and clinical trials when, in August 1989 at the age of 32, he was diagnosed with kidney cancer. Surgery in October of that year revealed that his cancer had metastasized:

I looked very hard for a trial that would combine an adequate dose of interferon and interleukin-2. I knew that interleukin-2 had been shown to be highly promising in many other trials, so this was not like the typical Phase I trial where you're trying some brand new drug. The particular trial I found was Phase I only because they were using a different brand of interleukin than had been tested previously.

> I knew that Phase I trials were dose escalation trials, and I asked them what the different doses were. Looking at the doses, I realized from my reading that the first dose cohort would be 50 percent of what they were guessing would be the Phase II dose, the second dose cohort would be at the probable Phase II dose, and the third would be 50 percent higher. I asked which one I would be in, and it turned out, fortunately, that I would be in the third one. I wanted to get a really, really high dose. If I had been in the first dose cohort, I would have walked, but I probably would have stayed for the second one.

> The end point of the trial was not efficacy. The end point was setting the dose. But I knew that it was a trial that had some substantial potential for being efficacious. In most Phase I trials, the first people in the trial get too low a dose. You don't even know if the stuff works in most cases, and then you get an amount which is almost certainly not enough to make it work even if it does work. If you are hoping for efficacy, you should find out where they are in the dose escalation and make sure you're not first.

In addition to determining a treatment's MTD, the investigators will want to know how the human body processes the drug. This is known as the treatment's pharmacokinetics. Some drugs pass through the body very quickly. Others are retained in the liver or the kidneys or in fatty deposits. The body's own enzymes frequently metabolize the drug, transforming it into one or more other chemical compounds. These metabolites might themselves exert separate therapeutic or toxic effects. Patients enrolled in Phase I trials can expect many of their bodily fluids to be sampled quite a few times each day for pharmacokinetic analysis.

Some experts in the ethics of clinical trials are critical of the conduct of some Phase I cancer trials.[5] Their studies have revealed that patients considering Phase I trials are often misinformed, led to believe that the trial is intended to assess not only toxicity, but also efficacy. It's easy to see how this can happen. The patient is not the only one looking for hope in what might seem to be a hopeless situation. The investigators also have high hopes for the treatment they've designed, even though they're well aware that it's in the most preliminary stage of human testing.

In a survey of 30 cancer patients who had decided to enter a Phase I trial, 85 percent indicated that they entered the trial because of the possibility of therapeutic benefits. However, only 22 percent of the group actually expected to receive that benefit, an indication that in that trial, at least, most patients correctly understood that the probability of receiving some personal benefit was low.[6] In another survey of 37 cancer patients who enrolled in a Phase I trial, 70 percent indicated that they had enrolled to get the best medical care, not out of altruism.[7]

Some people close to the cancer clinical trial scene believe that it's permissible for investigators to communicate—and for patients to expect—therapeutic intent in a Phase I trial, even if there might not be a strong probability that the experimental treatment will be effective. And some Phase I trial designs are being changed so there are more opportunities for the patients to benefit. One example is the increased use of intra-patient escalation so that the first patients in the trial don't only get the lowest dose. They would be put on the higher dose if other patients can tolerate that dose. In addition, Phase I trial protocols often specify that a patient who seems to be benefiting from the treatment can continue receiving it even after the trial concludes.

Advantages of Phase I trials

Following are some of the advantages of participating in a Phase I clinical trial:[8]

- It's a chance to receive a treatment that might be better than anything else out there years before it hits the market.

- Although its toxicity in humans is unknown, the treatment has already been tested extensively in the laboratory, in the test tube, and on animals. The investigators will have a good estimate of the proper human dose and an idea of its side effects. In fact, the substance may have already been tested in humans for other illnesses, so its toxic effects might be relatively well understood.

- Unlike Phase II trials, Phase I trials do not require measurable disease. This term refers to tumors whose size can be easily measured, such as most nodules in the lung. Many cancers, such as kidney or prostate cancer that have metastasized to the bone, are not considered to be measurable, although they might be evaluable.

- Even though Phase I trials are not intended to establish efficacy, if the treatment seems to be working, you most likely will be able to continue treatment even after the end of the trial.

- Phase I trials are never randomized; all participants receive the experimental treatment.

- Even if the treatment does not work for you personally, you might take comfort in knowing that your participation in the trial will help other cancer patients down the road, and it will also help the advancement of medical science.

Disadvantages of Phase I trials

Before deciding to enter a Phase I clinical trial, you should also be aware of some of the potential disadvantages of participation:

- Phase I trials are meant to test a substance's toxicity and not whether it works on cancer.

- You might be among the first humans to be given this treatment. It may have serious side effects, possibly leading to serious illness or even permanent damage.

- The treatment might be ineffective against your cancer, or it might be no better than standard treatments.

- You may be given too low a dose for it to be effective.

- Phase I trials tend to be shorter than Phase II and III trials. You might therefore not receive the treatment for a long enough time for it to be fully effective.

- Because Phase I trials are typically conducted at a single location, you might have to travel long distances for treatment.

Phase II

The most important thing to know about Phase II trials is that although they are intended to determine whether a treatment is effective against cancer, they cannot determine whether the new treatment is any better than the standard treatment. Moreover, there's no assurance that the treatment will work at all; fewer than half the treatments tested in Phase II end up being tested in Phase III. On top of that, even if the new treatment does turn out to show some effect, it might be no better—and it might even be worse—than standard treatments.

Just because a treatment has passed its Phase I toxicity testing, there's no assurance that it's completely safe. To begin with, as all people with cancer are certainly aware, most cancer treatments are inherently toxic. Remember that Phase I studies involve only a small number of patients; if a certain side effect occurs in only one in a hundred patients, it may well be noticed first in a larger Phase II trial.

On the other hand, some people regard Phase II trials as the best avenue for cancer patients considering a clinical trial. Lydia Cunningham Rising, a Detroit-based patient advocate who has advised more than 500 cancer patients on clinical trials, gives the following advice:

> *If you qualify for more than one clinical trial, all things being equal, I would take the Phase II. Phase I is obviously more experimental. It's a toxicity trial, so there's a greater chance for adverse side effects and less of a chance of a therapeutic effect. And when*

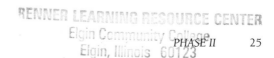

you go into a Phase III trial, you have the chance of being randomized.

Lydia Rising's first lesson in clinical trials was a baptism by fire in 1984, when her first husband, Joe Cunningham, was diagnosed with a rare, malignant brain tumor called primary central nervous system lymphoma:

Joe was basically told to go home and get his affairs in order, but he is alive and well today—14 years later—due to an experimental treatment he received 2,000 miles away from home.

Despite being assured by the physicians at her community medical center that Joe's tumor was inoperable, Lydia persisted in finding a neurosurgeon at the Mayo Clinic who was perfecting a new surgical technique. This operation was successful in removing Joe's "inoperable" tumor.

Then, just four months later, after a course of radiation therapy, Joe's cancer returned. Desperate to find some other avenue to a cure, Lydia began researching the medical literature. She learned that chemotherapy for brain cancers is often ineffective because of the blood-brain barrier, a protective mechanism found in the brain's blood vessels that keeps out most foreign substances. In addition to protecting the brain from bacteria, viruses, and poisons, the blood-brain barrier unfortunately also prevents many healing medications from getting through. But Lydia also learned about Dr. Edward Neuwelt of the Oregon Health Science University, who was experimenting with a technique called barrier disruption.

Dr. Neuwelt found a way to temporarily break down the blood-brain barrier, allowing chemotherapy to reach the tumor. His studies had just reached Phase II, and Joe enrolled in the trial:

My husband was the tenth person in the world to have this treatment. Within a month after treatments started, 90 percent of the tumor was gone, and by the end of the year, there was no trace of it.

Now, thirteen years later, Joe remains cancer free—not bad for a man who was given less than a five percent chance of surviving five years.[9]

Phase II trials typically enroll 50 to 100 patients, and in most—but not all—Phase II cancer trials, there's no randomization. Moreover, patients are generally given a more thorough course of therapy than in phase I.

However, the requirements for entering a Phase II trial are often very strict because, for statistical rigor, the investigators want to test the treatment on a homogeneous group of patients with well-defined disease.

One of the criteria for most Phase II trials, in contrast to those of Phase I and Phase III, is that patients must have measurable disease. Steve Dunn explains:

> *In Phase II trials, the objective is to see what percentage*
> *of people have their tumors shrink and go away and how long*
> *they stay away. It turns out that in order to do that, you need a*
> *tumor you can measure the size of. That way, when it gets smaller*
> *you can tell.*

Unfortunately for some patients who want to participate in Phase II trials, some types of cancer—such as cancer that has metastasized to the bone—are not measurable:

> *If you're a patient with kidney cancer and you had a recurrence*
> *only in your bones, you might not be able to get into a Phase II*
> *trial. If it has spread to the lungs, though, and there are these*
> *measurable nodules, then you probably could get into a*
> *Phase II trial.*

If some lesions are measurable and others are not, you still have measurable disease. For example, if your kidney cancer has spread to both your bones and your lungs, it's likely that your lung lesions will be measurable. Also, the exact definition of the term "measurable" varies from trial to trial and might be quite technical. You shouldn't rule yourself out just because you think you might not have measurable disease. If you believe a certain trial is promising, let the investigators decide whether or not you qualify.

Advantages of Phase II trials

The following are some of the advantages of participating in a Phase II clinical trial:

- As with Phase I trials, it's a chance to receive a treatment that might be better than anything else out there years before it hits the market.

- Treatments in Phase II trials have passed Phase I toxicity testing, and the maximally tolerated dose has already been determined. This generally means that you'll be given the highest dose that had acceptable toxicity.

- Phase II cancer trials are usually not randomized.

- Phase II trials tend to last longer than Phase I trials, increasing the likelihood that you'll experience a therapeutic effect.

- Even if the treatment does not work for you personally, you can take comfort in knowing that your participation in the trial will help other cancer patients down the road, and it will also help the advancement of medical science.

Disadvantages of Phase II trials

Disadvantages of participation in a Phase II trial include the following:

- The treatment might be ineffective against your cancer, or it might be no more effective than standard treatments.

- Even though the treatment has passed Phase I toxicity testing, you might experience unexpected or serious side effects, including those that can lead to permanent damage.

- The inclusion and exclusion criteria are usually very strict.

- You will generally be eligible for Phase II trials only if you have measurable disease.

- A Phase II trial tends to last longer than a Phase I trial. It will likely require more clinic visits and a greater time commitment.

- Because Phase II trials are sometimes not multicenter trials, you might have to travel long distances for treatment.

Phase III

The most important thing to know about Phase III trials is that they are intended to see whether a new treatment is any better than the current standard treatments by making direct comparisons with those treatments. Sometimes, there are two standard treatments for a certain type of cancer, and a Phase III trial is conducted to decide treatment is better. A treatment might be better if more patients go into remission, if they stay in remission for a longer time, or if they suffer fewer side effects, compared to current treatments.

Although the goal in Phase II trials is to find a relatively homogeneous group of patients, Phase III investigators are looking for a more widely representative sample of the population. They will attempt to enroll hundreds or thousands of participants, preferably from all walks of life. As a consequence, inclusion and exclusion criteria might be less strict than in Phase II trials. Measurable disease, for example, is usually not required. Because many Phase III trials are multicenter trials, patients can be seen at medical centers in many parts of the country, so travel may be less of a burden.

On the other hand, investigators will generally be looking for patients who are newly diagnosed and who have not yet received treatment for their cancer. Patients who have already received the standard or an experimental treatment might be excluded from Phase III trials.

Phase III trials tend to be much longer than Phase I and II trials because the investigators are often interested in keeping track of how well the participants do years into the future.

Most Phase III trials are randomized. In a simple Phase III trial, patients will be randomly assigned to receive the experimental treatment or the best available standard treatment. Often, however, the trial design may be more complex. Sometimes, there may be two or more versions of the experimental treatment for comparison to two or more versions of standard treatments. For that reason, it's very important for people considering Phase III trials to examine the trial's informed consent and protocol documents carefully to determine the chance of receiving experimental treatment.

Phase III trials are sometimes conducted in single- or double-blind fashion. As previously discussed, blinding is often pointless in cancer clinical trials; nevertheless, investigators conduct blinded studies whenever possible.

Larry Sands (not his real name) had a typical phase III experience soon after he was diagnosed with prostate cancer at the age of 45:

> I was having some obstructive urinary problems. I'm a physician's assistant, and at my age, I didn't think it was anything more serious than benign prostatic hypertrophy. My doctor drew blood for a PSA [prostate specific antigen] test, and it came back at 45, which is pretty high. Assuming that it was prostatitis, I took antibiotics for a month, but it rose to 47.

Larry's urologist diagnosed his problem as a moderately aggressive adenocarcinoma and recommended a radical prostatectomy. But when the surgeon went in, he discovered that the cancer had spread to Larry's lymph nodes, so he didn't remove the prostate:

> When he woke me up, he told me that the cancer had already spread, that I had three to five years to live, and that I should go home and come back to see him in three months. I didn't think that was really logical, considering my age. I wanted to pursue

*treatment more aggressively. I looked for a clinical trial because
there was no approved therapy for my cancer, at least until I got
into bone pain.*

*I went to my local oncologist, and she had a list of clinical trials.
I went to the M.D. Anderson Cancer Center, which wasn't far from
where I lived. They looked at my pathology slides and randomized
me into a Phase III clinical trial.*

*One group received a relatively complex regimen of chemothera-
py, and the other group just got watchful waiting and standard
hormonal therapy since there was no standard chemotherapy for
the type of cancer I had. Fortunately, I was randomized into the
chemotherapy group. If I had been randomized into the other
group, I would have found another protocol. I wasn't willing to sit
and wait and do nothing.*

During the course of the trial, Larry's PSA dropped to undetectable
levels and stayed there for almost two years. However, his PSA
recently started rising again, and Larry was diagnosed with a rare
sarcoma of the prostate. Despite this setback, Larry does not regret
participating in the clinical trial:

*I think it worked. The treatment may or may not have convert-
ed this adenocarcinoma into a sarcoma. The sarcoma may have
been there to start with. There's just no way to tell. But sarcoma
does have standard chemo protocols, and I just finished a round of
chemotherapy.*

Advantages of Phase III trials

The following are some of the advantages of participating in a Phase
III clinical trial:

- It's a chance to receive a treatment that might be better than
  anything else out there a year or two before it hits the market.

- Treatments in Phase III trials have passed Phase I toxicity
  testing, and Phase II testing has proven them to be at least
  somewhat effective.

- Although you might be randomized to one of the standard treatment arms, the Data Safety and Monitoring Board will switch you to the experimental treatment during the course of the trial if it turns out to be significantly more effective.

- Similarly, if the experimental treatment proves to be less effective, patients in that arm of the study will be switched to the standard treatment.

- Inclusion and exclusion criteria for Phase III trials are generally less strict than in earlier phases. Measurable disease is often not a requirement.

- Because Phase III trials are generally multicenter trials, you might have to travel a shorter distance for treatments.

- Even if the treatment does not work for you personally, you can take comfort in knowing that your participation in the trial will help other cancer patients down the road, and it will also help the advancement of medical science.

Disadvantages of Phase III trials

Some of the disadvantages of participating in a Phase III clinical trial follow:

- Many people do not want to take the chance of being randomized into a standard treatment arm, and with blinded trials, many people do not like being kept in the dark about which treatment they're receiving.

- Even if you are randomized into the experimental arm of the study, the experimental treatment might be no better than the standard treatment, and it might be worse.

- Phase III is the first time the treatment is being given to a large and diverse group of patients. Adverse side effects that were not seen in earlier phases are likely to show up during Phase III trials.

- Phase III trials are often reserved for newly diagnosed patients who have not previously received treatment.

Phase IV

If a new cancer treatment proves safe in Phase I, effective in Phase II, and better than standard treatments in Phase III, the treatment's sponsor (generally a pharmaceutical company) will apply to the US Food and Drug Administration (FDA) for approval to market the treatment widely.

If the FDA grants marketing approval, it may sometimes do so under the condition that the pharmaceutical company keeps track of how the treatment performs in the general population. This is known as post-marketing or Phase IV testing. Sometimes, the pharmaceutical company will conduct a Phase IV study on its own, even when not required to do so by the FDA.

Many Phase IV studies are not clinical trials in the same sense that earlier phases are. Some Phase IV studies are conducted informally, and patients who participate in Phase IV often have no idea that they're part of a research study. In these casual studies, no one is asked to sign an informed consent form, for example. (This is not true of all Phase IV studies, some of which are conducted quite formally, with the informed consent of all participants.)

In casual Phase IV studies, the drug company asks physicians to keep track of how their patients receiving the new treatment are doing. They're asked to report any adverse reactions, for example. Sometimes, pharmaceutical companies encourage physicians to submit these reports by paying them a fee for each report that's sent in.[10]

Although a full discussion of Phase IV studies is beyond the scope of this book, some critics of the pharmaceutical industry charge that Phase IV studies tend to be less about the advancement of clinical knowledge and more about the advancement of the pharmaceutical companies' marketing campaigns.[11] Critics charge that companies sponsor these trials to get physicians used to prescribing—and patients used to taking—their new drugs. Many Phase IV studies seem to be poorly designed from a scientific point of view, and their results rarely appear in scientific literature.

CHAPTER THREE

Clinical Trial Ethics

MANY PEOPLE ARE RELUCTANT to participate in clinical trials because they feel a sense of distaste for the idea of being experimented on, for being treated as if they were human guinea pigs. You've probably heard about the horrific medical experiments conducted on unwilling participants in Nazi concentration camps during World War II.[1] You may also have heard about the shameful Tuskegee experiment, in which 400 African-American men with syphilis were left untreated for decades—even after a cure for syphilis became available—so that scientists could study the natural course of the disease.[2] Those historical incidents along with several others—not to mention uncounted numbers of mad-scientist movies—have made many people wary of participating in clinical trials.

Fortunately, it's extremely rare these days for research subjects to be treated badly. Past abuses have led to the development of strict ethical codes for the conduct of clinical trials. Since the mid-1960s, participants in clinical trials have been the beneficiaries of strong ethical, legal, and procedural protections. But that doesn't mean that all ethical questions surrounding clinical trials have been solved or that you can assume that all clinical trials are conducted in an exemplary fashion. Moreover, you'll want to understand some of the competing ethical principles involved in clinical trials, and you'll want to know how designers of clinical trials decide what's in the patient's best interests and what constitutes an ethical clinical trial.

This chapter examines the checkered history of clinical trials and discusses the development of the ethical codes that are currently in force. Examples describe the ethical responsibilities of investigators and of patients. Also included is a discussion on what to do and how to complain if you encounter an ethical problem—or any other kind of problem—while participating in a clinical trial.

Early history

Human beings have probably been conducting clinical trials since before the dawn of civilization. The first person who realized that a wound that's cleaned and wrapped heals better than one that's left open and dirty conducted a kind of primitive clinical trial.

A passage in the Old Testament even describes a clinical trial. The first chapter of the Book of Daniel tells what happens after Nebuchadnezzar, king of Babylon, conquered Israel.

The king ordered that several Jewish youths be brought to his palace for three years, where they would be fed and taught just like his own children. Among the youths was Daniel, who did not want to defile himself by eating the king's meat or drinking his wine. He proposed to Melzar, the king's head eunuch, that they be allowed to eat "pulse" (a term referring to peas and beans) and to drink water instead. But Melzar feared Nebuchadnezzar's wrath if the Jewish youths grew sick. So Daniel suggested an experiment:

> "Prove thy servants, I beseech thee, ten days; and let them give us pulse to eat and water to drink. Then let our countenances be looked upon before thee, and the countenance of the children that eat of the portion of the king's meat: and as thou seest, deal with thy servants." So he consented to them in this manner and proved them ten days. And at the end of ten days, their countenances appeared fairer and fatter in flesh than all the children which did

eat the portion of the king's meat. Thus Melzar took away the portion of their meat, and the wine that they should drink; and gave them pulse.[3]

Clinical trials are also discussed in ancient Greek, Roman, and Arab medical works, but it wasn't until the 12th and 13th centuries A.D. that any ethical codes regarding human experimentation were written down.[4] Moses Maimonides (1135–1204), the Jewish physician, philosopher, and Rabbi of Cairo, taught that physicians should seek to help individual patients and should not use them merely as a way of learning new facts. Roger Bacon (1214–1294), the English scientist, philosopher, and Franciscan monk, noted that it was difficult for the physician to conduct experiments on living humans "because of the nobility of the material in which he works; for that body demands that no error be made in operating upon it...."

It wasn't until the 18th and 19th centuries that clinical trials became a fairly common way of testing new medical treatments. Often, physicians would test potential remedies on themselves or on close friends and relatives. In developing the smallpox vaccine in 1789, the English physician Edward Jenner first tried inoculating his own son, then just one year old, with swinepox in the hope that the milder form of the disease that affected pigs would prevent the child from developing a far more serious human disease. Unfortunately, Jenner's son caught smallpox anyway. Several months later, Jenner inoculated a neighbor's child with cowpox, followed a week later with an injection of smallpox. The child didn't get the disease, proving that vaccination worked.

The famous French physician Louis Pasteur (1822–1895) was a brilliant practitioner of human experimentation, and he was also keenly aware of the ethical implications of his work. In one of his lines of research, he worked for many years using animal experiments to develop an antidote for rabies, and in 1884, he finally had a remedy that he thought would be highly effective. Yet he agonized about when and whether to try his antidote on a person. Only after being begged by the mother of a nine-year-old boy who had been bitten by a rabid dog, and after consulting with two colleagues who assured him that the child would certainly die without treatment, was he persuaded to administer the antidote. Feeling great anxiety, Pasteur gave the child twelve inoculations. The boy lived.

During the course of the 19th century, larger and more organized clinical trials became increasingly typical in medicine. Ethical protection of research subjects also became part of Anglo-American common law, which carefully distinguished between science and quack medicine and which regarded clinical trials as legitimate—providing the researcher had the participant's agreement.

With the increasing prevalence of clinical trials came some ethically questionable practices, however. While working in Panama on his groundbreaking work on yellow fever, the American physician Walter Reed (1851–1902) sought volunteers among American soldiers. These soldiers would allow themselves to be bitten by mosquitoes, which Reed believed (correctly, as it turned out) were the source of the infection. In seeking subjects, Reed offered his volunteers the princely sum of $100 in gold for allowing themselves to be bitten, and those who actually contracted yellow fever were given a bonus of another $100. But he exaggerated greatly while recruiting volunteers. He enticed people to join the experiment by stating that a case of yellow fever endangers life only "to a certain extent," when in fact the disease could often be fatal. And he also said that it would be "entirely impossible" for non-volunteers living in Panama to avoid the infection, when in fact many people did not catch the disease, even though it was epidemic.

In the years before World War II, some of the world's most prominent physicians, including George Sternberg, the Surgeon General of the United States, believed that it was permissible to conduct experiments on vulnerable populations. Infants, condemned prisoners, and people who lived in large state institutions for the mentally retarded were frequently used in medical experimentation, including experiments that were clearly not designed to be therapeutic. To mention just one shocking example, orange juice was withheld from orphans at the Hebrew Infant Asylum of New York City so doctors could study the development of scurvy. Few if any of these experiments were regarded as unethical at the time, and the investigators were hardly criticized for their practices.

The Nuremberg Code

In his article on the history of human research, David J. Rothman describes World War II as the "transforming event" in the conduct of clinical trials.[5] Although the odious experiments performed by the Nazis on concentration-camp inmates have received the most attention in that regard—and were the only ones to be prosecuted after the war—it's important to remember that under the pressure of the wartime emergency, the Allies also conducted medical experiments that would be regarded as highly unethical today.

The Nazi experiments are almost too horrible to describe.[6] Inmates were placed in decompression chambers to simulate the effects of extremely high altitudes. They were plunged into icy water to see how long downed pilots could survive. They were injected with toxins and with infectious agents, including typhus. They were intentionally given mutilating wounds. Almost all the subjects of these experiments died in the course of the research. One of the many awful aspects of this history is that the majority of these studies were entirely without scientific merit.

Out of this horror came the first formalized set of ethical rules for the conduct of human experimentation. In the aftermath of the war, the Nuremberg Tribunal prosecuted the perpetrators and in 1946 developed a set of ethical principles that have come to be known as the Nuremberg Code. The Nuremberg Code is printed in its entirety in Appendix B, *Critical Public Documents*.

In remarkably clear and definitive language, the Code sets out ten ethical principles for the conduct of clinical trials. The first is the most important: "The voluntary consent of the human subject is absolutely essential." Moreover, this consent must be obtained "without the intervention of any element of force, fraud, deceit, duress, over-reaching, or other ulterior form of constraint or coercion...."

The Code directs researchers to ensure that experiments on humans are well designed, conducted by qualified personnel based on the results of animal experimentation, and have a degree of risk commensurate with the humanitarian importance of the problem to be solved. In other words, the Code says that you can conduct an experiment with potentially dangerous side effects if you're trying to cure a deadly disease such as cancer, but not if you're only trying to cure the common cold.

The Code also gives the participant the right to leave the trial at any time, "if he has reached the physical or mental state where continuation of the experiment seems to him to be impossible."

Continuing abuses

Despite the clear language of the Nuremberg Code, and despite the fact that it is regarded by many as the gold standard for the conduct of clinical trials, it does have a number of problems. For one thing, if it's interpreted literally, the Code seems to prohibit any research involving children or the mentally incompetent, such as people with Alzheimer's disease. That's because children and the mentally incompetent do not have "the legal capacity to give consent," in the words of the Nuremberg Code. The Code makes no provision for consent by parents or legal guardians.[7]

Perhaps the biggest problem with the Nuremberg Code is that although it had some moral force, it did not have the force of law in the United States, and its provisions were widely ignored for at least twenty years.[8] Rothman writes that from the point of view of most American investigators, "[T]he Code had nothing to do with science and everything to do with Nazis. The guilty parties were seen less as doctors than as Hitler's henchmen." This left American physicians free to conduct clinical trials simply in accordance with their consciences and with virtually no oversight or regulation.

During the postwar years, the American Medical Association developed a research code, and the World Medical Association issued the Helsinki Declaration with detailed rules for human experimentation. Although these documents were the subject of a great deal of discussion in the medical community, neither proved to have much influence on the conduct of clinical trials.

Then, in June 1966, the tide turned. Henry K. Beecher, an anesthesiologist at Harvard Medical School, published a highly influential article entitled "Ethics and Clinical Research" in the *New England Journal of Medicine*.[9] In his article, he listed no fewer than 22 clinical trials that appeared to be highly unethical, in which researchers risked their patients' lives without fully informing them of the dangers and without obtaining their permission.

In one of these cases, investigators fed live hepatitis virus to mentally retarded residents of Willowbrook, a state institution in New York. In another case, investigators injected live cancer cells into senile patients at the Brooklyn Jewish Chronic Disease hospital to observe their immunological responses. In neither case were the experimental subjects properly informed of the dangers of the research. In neither case did the research have any potential therapeutic value to the patients under study.

Then, in 1970, came the revelation of the Tuskegee experiment. Starting in 1930 and continuing for four long decades, investigators began examining—but not treating—a group of 400 African-American men who had contracted syphilis. The researchers were interested in watching the natural course of the disease as it developed.

In 1930, the existing treatments for syphilis were complex and not very effective, so the researchers felt they were justified in not treating the men. But what could the researchers have been think-ing when they took steps to make sure the men would not be drafted into the army, where they would have received treatment? And how did the researchers rationalize leaving the men untreated even after penicillin became widely available in 1945? Penicillin is a highly effective cure for syphilis. In fact, many of the men were left untreated until the scandal was uncovered in 1970.

The modern era

The uproar over the Tuskegee experiment and the Beecher article led directly to substantive changes in the way clinical trials were run in this country. The National Institutes of Health (NIH) quickly established rules requiring that committees called Institutional Review Boards (IRBs) be set up at each facility con-ducting clinical trials. IRBs were charged with conducting peer review of proposed research involving human beings. For the first time, individual investigators were not permitted to decide for themselves whether their research was ethical. Instead, it had to pass the muster of their colleagues.

The FDA, for its part, issued regulations that concentrated more on consumer protection. These regulations were the first to require that investigators obtain fully informed consent from potential subjects.

The US Congress followed in 1973 by creating the National Commission for the Protection of Human Subjects of Biomedical and Behavioral Research. Made up of eleven members, only a minority of whom were researchers (the remainder were experts in such fields as law, ethics, philosophy, and theology), the National Commission in 1979 issued a highly influential document known as the Belmont Report. The Belmont Report is included in its entirety in Appendix B. Its language is clear and eloquent and applies to how clinical trials are designed today.

The Belmont Report lays out three basic ethical principles for the conduct of clinical trials:

- **Respect for Persons.** Individuals should be regarded as autonomous agents, and their opinions and choices should be respected. Some people, such as children or individuals with mental incapacities, are not fully capable of self-determination, and those people should be subject to special protection.

- **Beneficence.** The Belmont Report's definition of beneficence goes beyond its common meaning, which covers acts of charity or kindness. The National Commission regarded beneficence as an actual obligation, involving two rules: 1) do no harm, and 2) maximize benefits and minimize harms.

- **Justice.** The benefits of research should be distributed fairly.

In applying those principles, the report's authors recommended that consideration be given to three requirements:

- **Informed consent.** To provide fully informed consent, a potential research subject must first be given full information about the research project. Second, that information must be presented in a comprehensible way, taking into account the patient's intellectual capacities. If these capacities are limited, as they are in children or people who are mentally disabled, the consent of responsible third parties must be sought. However, if this guardian agrees to the research but the patient objects, this objection must be respected, unless the study involves therapy that's unavailable outside the research setting. Third, the consent must be truly voluntary and free from coercion and undue influence. Coercion occurs when there is a threat of harm. "You're going to die if you don't agree to participate," is an improper, coercive statement. Undue influence occurs through the offer of an excessive or inappropriate reward. "If you participate in this clinical trial, we'll cure your cancer," is an example of undue influence.

- **Assessment of risks and benefits.** The dangers of any clinical trial must not exceed its potential benefits. Both the researcher and the IRB must explicitly consider not only the risks to a particular research subject, but also the risks to the subject's family and to society at large.

- **Selection of subjects.** There must be fair procedures for the selection of research subjects. Investigators must not select certain patients merely because they like them. Conversely, investigators must not seek out undesirable people, such as prisoners, for especially risky experiments.

The federal regulations setting all the rules for the conduct of clinical trials were revised most recently in 1991. They are part of the Code of Federal Regulations, Title 45, which deals with public welfare. The relevant section is Part 46, "Protection of Human Subjects." Although these regulations are too lengthy to print here, it's a good idea to take a look at them, especially if you suspect a violation of the rules. You can find the full text in public libraries or online at the site *http://www.med.umich.edu/irbmed/FederalDocuments/hhs/HHS45CFR46.html.*

Adherence to these regulations has significantly improved protections for research subjects. Clinical trials are conducted far more ethically and are far safer now than they were 30 years ago. But this certainly does not mean that every ethical problem has been solved. On the contrary, the elimination of gross abuses tends to highlight more subtle ethical problems. The following sections discuss some of the ethical dilemmas that confront investigators and patients during the conduct of clinical trials.

The investigator's responsibilities

The investigator conducting a clinical trial has awesome medical and ethical responsibilities, some of which are in conflict. If she is both a physician and a researcher, as are most people conducting cancer clinical trials, she must reconcile her responsibility to give each individual patient the best possible treatment with her responsibility to conduct scientifically valid experiments to advance the boundaries of medical knowledge. Harold Y. Vanderpool, professor in the history and philosophy of medicine at the University of Texas Medical Branch at Galveston, explains:

> The investigators' ethical responsibility has primarily to do with their finding an ethically justified balance between the benefits of their research for patients now and in the future against a respect for the persons and choices of the patients. They need to be responsible students of research ethics and not see ethics as something that gets in the way of effective research.

Nowhere is this conflict more evident than when your physician offers you the opportunity to participate in a clinical trial for which she's an investigator. Steve Dunn comments:

> There is this conflict of interest between patients and the people doing the research. People doing the research need to get valid data, and patients need to get the best possible treatment. Sometimes these coincide exactly, and sometimes they don't.

Dr. Vanderpool discusses the issue of trust:

> One of the biggest problems is the degree to which patients trust their physicians and the degree to which physicians, failing to distinguish between the ethics of clinical practice and the ethics of research, offer "Trust me" statements. There are important degrees of trust between doctors and patients, and that's good. But if that same level of trust is there for the researcher, then the patient will assume, "Well, the doctor is just here for my own health interests," when the research protocol says the doctor is there fundamentally to advance medical knowledge. Cancer patients are in a one-down psychological position. They have to trust their doctors. They want a cure. They need a cure. They dare not risk any kind of a personal distance or alienation from the physician-researcher. So they're very much inclined to do what the researcher wants and to accede to the requests of researchers.

This conflict often comes to a head during the informed consent process. When your doctor, who presumably has an intimate knowledge of your medical condition, recommends that you consider a clinical trial, your first inclination will be to sign on the dotted line without giving much thought to the possible negative consequences of participating. One participant remembers:

> When you're faced with, "This, that, or the other thing may happen," versus "You have cancer. It's going to kill you," which way do you go? It's not a hard decision. At least, that was my feeling then.

The responsible physician-researcher will be conscious of his power—and his patient's vulnerability—in this situation. Dr. David Jablons of the University of California, San Francisco, describes what he does when faced with a patient who's not asking enough questions, a patient who says, "Doc, whatever you say is fine with me. I don't even want to read the document. Just show me where to sign."

> I basically say, "No. I really want you to go home, spend a week, spend a weekend, get some more opinions about this, and think about it." You don't want anyone signing on just because they're desperate. The other problem is that people who are running clinical trials are by definition optimistic. You can't spend twenty hours a day doing this stuff and trying to push the frontier without believing at some point that it's going to help. That optimism obviously is contagious, and the patients get caught up in that. I try to objectively present what the pros and cons are. I say, "There's no guarantee that this is going to make a difference, no guarantee that you will get a response, and depending on how the trial is written, no guarantee that you'll even get the drug, if you get randomized into the placebo arm."

Dr. Vanderpool warns against another pitfall:

> I think physicians need to be aware of the degree to which some cancer patients are in an almost coercive environment in the

hospital. If the patient goes on protocol, the patient will get a special team, special attention, regular checking and be part of an esprit de corps. If they don't go on protocol and their cancers are terminal, they're going to get threadbare, less enthusiastic, less professionalized care. So I think it's important that physicians not sell their protocols by saying, "Now, if you enroll in this, we'll be able to give you all this attention."

Adding to the conflict within the single person who is both physician and researcher are the financial and professional rewards available to successful investigators.[10] Many pharmaceutical companies pay physicians a fee for each patient recruited to a clinical trial. (Such payments are rare for trials sponsored by federal agencies such as the National Cancer Institute, although NCI cooperative groups do pay the institution for data management.) At some medical institutions, physicians are required to attract enough money through grants and fees to subsidize all or part of their salaries. In other institutions, physicians pocket these fees for patient recruitment as a bonus above and beyond their regular salaries. In either case, there is a direct relationship between the physician's paycheck and the number of patients she recruits to her clinical trials.

Then, there are the professional rewards. You're probably familiar with the phrase "publish or perish." Physician-researchers at academic medical centers are expected to publish scientific papers, and if they don't, their careers might be derailed. One sure route to publication is to conduct clinical trials. Adding to the pressure to recruit patients is the tradition in multicenter trials for the investigator who has recruited the largest number of patients to be listed as primary author of the scientific paper announcing the study's results. Therefore, there's at least an indirect relationship between a physician's professional advancement and the number of patients she recruits to her clinical trials.

Please do not misunderstand: this doesn't imply that physician-researchers are crooks or con men out to trick innocent patients into second-rate clinical trials in order to collect a bounty of financial and professional rewards. On the contrary, the vast majority of physicians participating as investigators in clinical trials clearly conduct themselves with the highest level of personal and professional ethics. They are mindful of their potential conflicts of interest, and they take conscious steps to avoid these conflicts.

Nevertheless those conflicts are there, and as a patient, you too must be conscious of them. What does this mean on an operational level? Perhaps it means that you should get a second opinion if your physician suggests you participate in a clinical trial that she's personally involved in. Perhaps it means that you should look into other therapies and clinical trials (using the techniques in Chapter 4, *How to Find Clinical Trials*), even if your physician presents a convincing case that her trial offers you the best chance. You may independently come to the same conclusion, or you might find another avenue that offers even more hope.

Dr. Vanderpool talks about the responsibility of those who are supporting and sponsoring trials:

> *I think medical centers have the responsibility not to place monetary pressure on their researchers and their departments in such a way that institutional self-interest outweighs ethical responsibility. Sponsors should avoid placing restrictions, pressures, or temptations toward self-interest on researchers. That could compromise the rights of patients. I think the sponsors themselves should care about such pressures on the researchers and shouldn't hype the prospects of this drug beyond an accurate reading of what they've discovered up to the point it's being used. I think they have to be honest, and they have to be aware that the pressures they might place on researchers or the rewards they might give to researchers might compromise the protections and rights of patients.*

These potential conflicts of interest mean that you should take a very careful look at the informed consent document (see Chapter 7, *Evaluating a Clinical Trial*), you should ask a lot of questions, and you should consider all your options carefully before agreeing to participate in any clinical trial. Don't just sign on the dotted line because you're scared, you like your doctor, and you're sure she has your best interests at heart. Sign on the dotted line after thoroughly informing yourself and convincing yourself that you're following the best possible course of action under the circumstances.

The patient's responsibilities

As a culture, we value altruism. Many of our heroes practice self-denial, and we regard selfishness as suspect. Therefore, it's important to know that as a patient, it is perfectly ethical for you to act with self-interest as your primary focus. You shouldn't be ashamed of searching out the best possible treatment or the most promising clinical trial. And you shouldn't be embarrassed to ask question after question in your effort to decide what's best to do in what may well be a life-threatening situation.

But how far does the ethical imperative toward personal survival go? Would it be permissible to lie in order to get into a trial or to use deception to get into the preferred arm of a trial? Is it wrong to have unrealistic hope? Is there an actual ethical obligation for people with cancer to participate in clinical trials? These are difficult questions, and the answers aren't always clear. Obviously, it isn't possible to consider every conceivable situation here, but let's examine several scenarios and discuss their ethical implications. Think carefully about any ethical dilemmas that present themselves during the course of your cancer treatment. Discuss them with trusted friends, relatives, and spiritual advisors. Many hospitals have experts in bioethics available for advice and consultation on these matters. And remember that reasonable, honorable, and ethical people often arrive at different solutions to ethical problems. It's not always easy to know what's right.

Scenario 1: Fudging the criteria

Let's say that you have cancer and you've identified a clinical trial that seems perfect; it's testing an exciting new treatment that you are convinced may lead to a cure. But let's say that you don't quite meet the inclusion criteria. Perhaps one of your lab results is just slightly worse than the acceptable values. Is it permissible for you to lie about those lab results or to have your personal physician lie to the investigator about them?

Dr. Vanderpool says that it's not permissible to lie in this situation. "It undermines the entire research enterprise. You could damn an entire line of research by doing that."

That's because a treatment that is actually effective on people who are moderately ill might be ineffective on people who are more seriously ill. If enough seriously ill people mask the severity of their condition in order to sneak into the trial, the treatment may seem less effective than it really is. It might be abandoned even though many people could have been helped by it. Because your deception could potentially deny an effective treatment to many others, it would be unethical to lie in this situation.

Scenario 2: Re-rolling the dice

What about the scenario discussed by Steve Dunn in the section on randomization in Chapter 2, *The Structure of Clinical Trials?* If you were randomized into the standard-treatment arm of a clinical trial, and you desperately wanted to receive the study medication, would it be ethical for you to drop out of the study at one location and use deception to enter the study at another in an effort to get a more favorable roll of the dice?

First of all, you should recognize that you might be mistaken about whether it would be better to receive the study medication. Clinical trials are conducted in order to figure out whether the study medication is better than the standard treatment. If the scientists already knew the answer to that question, there'd be no reason to conduct the trial.

Second, it is clearly ethical for you to drop out of a study at any time for any reason or for no reason. That's a right guaranteed to you in every document related to clinical trials, from the Nuremberg Code to the Belmont Report to federal regulations, and it is mentioned explicitly in every informed consent document.

But Dr. Vanderpool says that it would not be ethical for you to lie in order to get into the trial at another location. On the other hand, he says, you are under no obligation to tell the whole truth. If someone at the second site asks you whether you have ever been in a clinical trial before, you must answer honestly, revealing that you had been in this same trial at a different location and that you had dropped out. However, when you are asked why you dropped out, Dr. Vanderpool says that you wouldn't have to give all the reasons. You could just say something like, "I was just going through a time where I didn't want to continue in that trial, but upon second thought, I do want to get in it, and I have every expectation I'll stay."

It might be argued that re-rolling the dice like this might de-randomize the study. Patients with more aggressive personality traits, or ones more willing to take risks, might tend to accumulate in certain arms of the trial. According to Dr. Vanderpool, this theoretical possibility does not present an actual ethical problem. Randomization criteria typically depend on physical and not psychological traits. Psychological traits would enter the equation only if, for example, the patient had clinical depression for which he was taking medication. Moreover, it's up to the investigators to control the entry criteria so that their trial will be acceptably randomized. On top of that, there's no evidence that leaving and re-entering trials is a widespread practice. In fact, while researching this book, we were unable to identify a single patient willing to admit that he had tried this technique or a single investigator who knew of such an occurrence.

Scenario 3: Risky behavior

Let's assume that you have a type of cancer for which there is no good standard treatment, and the only clinical trial you can find is a Phase I trial. If you've read Chapter 2, you know that Phase I trials are risky and that they are not even intended to determine whether the experimental treatment works. They're only intended to determine how toxic it is and what the maximally tolerated dose would be.

If the investigators have been completely honest with you, as of course they should be, they would inform you that this trial had little chance of leading to a cure for you personally. In fact, studies show that only 4 to 6 percent of people enrolled in Phase I cancer trials show any response at all, and of course far fewer achieve complete remission.[11] However, despite those dismal odds, of the Phase I participants who were surveyed, 100 percent said they participated because of the possibility of benefit, 89 percent said it was because of the lack of a better option, 70 percent cited trust in their oncologist, and only 33 percent mentioned the possibility that their participation would help future patients.

The ethical question that emerges from these figures is this: is it wrong for a person to participate in a Phase I trial while underestimating the risks and overestimating the possibility of personal benefit? Dr. Vanderpool says:

> I think patients should have the right to go into a protocol even if they don't stand to benefit. They should be able to try long shots like entering Phase I protocols, where there's little therapeutic possibility. On the other hand, I can honestly say that when I'm in that situation, I'm going to scrutinize whether research is my

grounds for hope or whether going fishing or taking the time to
make things right with my family and getting palliative care is not
a better grounds for hope. There are certainly grounds for hope
outside of the doctors' purview and research protocols.

Scenario 4: An obligation to serve?

Some bioethicists believe that we may actually have an ethical duty
to participate in clinical trials.[12] The argument goes that as members
of society we have all benefited from the sacrifices of those who
have participated in clinical trials in the past, so we owe it to future
generations to participate in clinical trials ourselves.

Most ethicists would not agree with the strongest form of that argument. After all, they say, you can't be expected to incur obligations
as part of a social group if you never consented to become part of
that group. Suppose you lived in a high-crime area, and some of
your neighbors formed a block patrol. They couldn't force you to
participate in the patrol even though you are receiving the benefits
of the patrol. You didn't choose to receive those benefits so you
incur no duty.

On the other hand, bioethicist Arthur L. Caplan argues that if you
choose to receive medical care at a research hospital—presumably
because you desire the best, most advanced treatment available—
you might then incur an ethical obligation to serve as a research
subject. After all, most patients in research hospitals are presumed
to have an obligation to serve as subjects for teaching purposes.
Your physician will often bring along medical students, interns, or
residents to participate in your examination, diagnosis, and treatment. Caplan argues that when you willingly go to a research
hospital, you have consented to being part of a certain social cooperative, so you do incur a duty to serve. He adds that this is a
general obligation and that you would have no duty to serve as a
subject in any specific clinical trial. Informed consent would still
apply, and you wouldn't be compelled to participate in studies that
pose significant risks.

Caplan's view is not held by a majority of bioethicists, so you needn't fear being forced to participate in a clinical trial merely by choosing to receive care at an academic medical center. Dr. Vanderpool offers his opinion:

> Insofar as we and our loved ones will have received therapeutic benefit thanks to research in the past, there should be some sense of responsibility for participating. But I think it's faulty to put that in the form of an ethical obligation. I think the philosopher Immanuel Kant was correct when he said that acts of beneficence are "imperfect duties." A "perfect duty" is something that you should always do, but an "imperfect duty" is something about which you make a judgment call, and whether to benefit others is that judgment call. It's true that I should benefit others, but how much I should do this and how much self-sacrifice I should show is subject to all kinds of considerations. So I think it's very problematic to obligate patients who are sick with cancer to go into clinical trials.

Dr. Vanderpool suggests that you weigh the argument about obligation and duty along with all the other factors you'll be considering while making your decision about whether to participate in a clinical trial.

How to complain

If you're having any kind of problem with any aspect of a clinical trial, you should first try to resolve it by speaking with the trial's clinical research coordinator (CRC) or the investigator. Only in the unlikely event that they are unable to resolve the problem should you take a complaint to higher levels.

The general principle you should follow in complaining is to escalate slowly. Don't go straight to the head of a federal agency, because problems can often be resolved at the local level and a resolution at that level is likely to be concluded far more quickly than if you make it a federal case.

If the investigator or CRC can't solve the problem, go to the local Institutional Review Board. Sometimes the IRB will be a committee within the medical center hosting the trial, but sometimes the medical center or a pharmaceutical company will contract with a private IRB that might not even be located in the same city. Often you'll be able to find the IRB's telephone number on your informed consent document. If it's not there, ask the investigator for the phone number. Ask to speak with the chairperson of the IRB. Outline your complaint calmly and completely. Be clear about how you hope to have the complaint resolved.

When the trial is a multicenter trial, there will be one chief investigator for the whole trial, perhaps at a different institution than the one where you're receiving treatment. In the rare instance you're unable to resolve your complaint at the local level, you can take it to the study's chief investigator. Another alternative for studies sponsored by pharmaceutical companies is to complain to the director of research at that company. You should be able to obtain contact information for the chief investigator or the director of research from the investigator at your institution or the local IRB. Sometimes merely requesting that information will be enough to underscore how serious you regard the issue and will encourage the local investigator to resolve the problem.

If these techniques don't work, your next step should be to contact the Office for Protection from Research Risks (OPRR), which is part of the US Department of Health and Human Services. Although the OPRR is administratively part of the NIH, it has jurisdiction over all clinical trials in the US, even those that are not sponsored by the NIH and its member institutes. The OPRR is responsible for administering the regulations in the Code of Federal Regulations, Title 45, Part 46, "Protection of Human Subjects." The OPRR maintains an informative web site at *http://www.nih.gov:80/grants/oprr/oprr.htm*.

It's wise to submit any complaints to OPRR in writing, although telephone calls are accepted as well. When writing, be sure to specify the nature of your inquiry (e.g., general guidance on policy or allegations of noncompliance) and the nature of the research activity (e.g., a single-center trial, a multicenter trial, etc.). Specify the name of the trial and the investigator's name, and if it's a multi-center trial, name the particular Cooperative Oncology Group (COG) or Community Clinical Oncology Program (CCOP) that's administering it. (See Chapter 8, *Administration of Clinical Trials*, for more on the administration of clinical trials.) The OPRR requests that you write the appropriate acronym in the lower left of the envelope (e.g., Re:COG or Re:CCOP if it's a multicenter trial, or the name of the state in which the research is taking place if it's a single-center trial). This allows the office staff to quickly route your inquiry to the appropriate person. The address of OPRR is listed in Appendix A, *Resources*.

If your problem is primarily with a pharmaceutical company, another place to complain is the FDA. The first step is to contact one of the FDA's Consumer Complaint Coordinators. There's a Consumer Complaint Coordinator in every state, and some large states have more than one. You'll find a complete list of phone numbers at *http://www.fda.gov/opacom/backgrounders/problem.html*. If you still can't get satisfaction, contact James C. Morrison, the ombudsman for the FDA's Center for Drug Evaluation and Research (CDER). His address is listed in Appendix A.

CHAPTER FOUR

How to Find
Clinical Trials

THERE ARE MANY WAYS to find clinical trials, including asking your doctor, calling the National Cancer Institute, searching various Internet sites, perusing news media, and hiring research services. Unfortunately, none of these methods is completely comprehensive. For that reason, you should use several techniques simultaneously, and you might want to repeat your searches once a week because new clinical trials are announced all the time.

The first step in using any of these methods is to know your full diagnosis. It's not enough to know that you have adrenal cancer, for example. You'll need its full medical name, including its stage (for example, inoperable stage III adrenocortical carcinoma).

Secondly, you or someone close to you needs to learn everything possible about your cancer. If you have no medical background, this might seem like a hopeless task, but it's not. Patient advocate Lydia Cunningham Rising offers suggestions:

> I tell people that if they want to do this themselves, start with the basics. Start by reading patient-education materials, things from the library. If you're reasonably intelligent, you can educate yourself in a very narrow area of medicine. If you need to know about one type of lung cancer, you can learn enough about that one thing. Do a magazine search at the library, and focus on the popular literature. You can go to the various cancer organizations. They're a wonderful resource. Lots of them have a great deal of

patient-geared educational material. If you start with those things, you can work your way up. Very few people can go bouncing directly into the medical library. Usually, I recommend that someone other than the patient do this. If you're sick, you might not have the stamina, and there's also the problem of being detached. When you're the one that has to go through the pain and the suffering, it's difficult to be objective. It's still difficult if it's a family member, but less so. I tell people that you have to be objective and not emotional. That's the only way to figure it out.

Janet Twombly offers similar encouragement:

Read everything you can get your hands on, or have someone read it for you. Get as much background as you can. Know what your options are. There are always options. You have the option of not doing anything. You have the option of conventional treatment. You have to be committed to taking the leap of faith it takes to try something new.

It'll help if you can get your hands on a comprehensive medical dictionary. See *Taber's Cyclopedic Medical Dictionary,* Clayton L. Thomas, ed., (Philadelphia: F.A. Davis Co., 1997); it's geared toward the nursing profession and tends to have a good deal of practical information that other dictionaries lack. Other good medical dictionaries are *Stedman's Medical Dictionary,* Thomas Lathrop Stedman, ed., (Baltimore: Lippincott Williams & Wilkins, 1995) and *Dorland's Illustrated Medical Dictionary,* W. A. Newman Dorland, ed., (Troy, MO: W. B. Saunders Co., 1994). All three of these dictionaries are updated every few years, and you should always try to obtain the most recent edition.

It's beyond the scope of this book to provide detailed suggestions on how to research your medical condition. However, several excellent books are available on this subject. See *Cancer Cure: How To Find And Get The Best There Is* (formerly titled *If the President Had Cancer...*) by Gary Schine with Ellen Berlinsky, (New York: Kensington Books, 1994), and *Informed Decisions: The Complete*

Book of Cancer Diagnosis, Treatment, and Recovery by Gerald P. Murphy, MD, Lois B. Morris, and Dianne Lange, (New York: Viking Penguin Books, 1997).

The best time to look for clinical trials is immediately after you've been diagnosed—before undergoing any treatment. Many clinical trials will exclude you if you've already had surgery or chemotherapy. Your physician might be eager for you to start treatment right away, so speed is of the essence as you determine whether a clinical trial may provide a better alternative to standard therapies.

Please don't take this to mean that it's pointless to investigate clinical trials if you've already had some treatment. Previous treatment will not always exclude you, and some clinical trials are specifically designed for people who have already undergone certain therapies.

Your doctor

Your primary care physician or oncologist is the first person you should approach about clinical trials. Once she has outlined your prognosis and the available treatment options, be sure to ask if she thinks you should consider clinical trials and if there are any she recommends. According to Lydia Cunningham Rising:

> *The whole experience depends on the initial MD. If you have someone who's open to a clinical trial, and is willing to review material that you send, the process is so much easier. If you don't find somebody like that, the process is hell.*

Don't be surprised, however, if your doctor isn't aware of many clinical trials. Information about clinical trials tends not to spread to physicians who work outside of major academic medical centers. Even if she has an affiliation with a major medical center, your oncologist likely has patients with all different kinds of cancer, and she's unlikely to be equipped with comprehensive information about each one of the 1,500 or so clinical trials available for those different diagnoses.

If your physician does recommend a specific clinical trial, be sure to ask her why she thinks this one is your best shot. It may be that the trial she's recommending is one that she's personally involved in as an investigator. Although it might be a perfectly fine trial, remember the old saying, "When all you have is a hammer, everything looks like a nail." When presented with only a single choice, you would do well to use the techniques outlined in this chapter to determine whether there are any other possibilities. This may complicate your decision about treatment, but too much information is almost always better than too little. Steve Dunn offers his perspective:

I wouldn't fire my oncologist just because he offered me his trial and didn't tell me about every trial in the entire country, and I wouldn't fire my community oncologist because he didn't bring up clinical trials right away. However, once I brought up these other issues, if I didn't see some kind of cooperation and help, then I would fire him.

You might find your physician expressing coolness or even hostility at the very idea of a clinical trial. Lydia Cunningham Rising says:

There's a wide variation in attitude among physicians. Some basically won't refer anybody to a clinical trial. They're not sure it's going to work, and they don't want to refer their patients to something that might make them worse. And some doctors have the attitude, "Why waste the last months of your life running around from hospital to hospital trying clinical trials? Why don't you just go home and be with the people you love?" Their personal views interfere.

Another patient advocate, Nancy Oster, suggests, "If you have a doctor that's really, really against it, and you feel really, really strongly, then you should probably find another doctor."

After investigating clinical trials, you may well decide not to pursue this avenue. But that should be your decision to make, and you should make it only after you have all the information and you've considered all the options. If your doctor won't help, just inform her that you intend to look into clinical trials on your own.

The National Cancer Institute

The National Cancer Institute (NCI) is a US government agency, the largest of the seventeen institutes that comprise the National Institutes of Health (NIH), which in turn is part of the Department of Health and Human Services. The NCI is the nation's premier center for cancer research. It sponsors both basic research and clinical trials, conducted at its Bethesda, Maryland, campus and at hundreds of other institutions around the country. A darling of Congress ever since President Richard Nixon declared the War on Cancer in 1971, the NCI's projected annual budget in fiscal year 1999 was a generous $2.93 billion. You'll find a great deal of information about cancer and the NCI on its main web page at *http://www.nci.nih.gov/*.

The NCI also provides a wonderful aid to the cancer community called the Cancer Information Service, whose toll-free number is (800) 4-CANCER. When you call that number, you'll be connected to an understanding, compassionate, and knowledgeable person who can give you a great deal of information about cancer in general and your specific cancer in particular. They have many brochures, videos, and other materials, most of which they'll send you at no charge. Be sure to ask them to send you their latest catalog, which has a complete list of available publications.

Best of all, the nice people at the Cancer Information Service will conduct a customized search of the PDQ database (described more fully in the next section) for you. They'll send you detailed information about most if not all the NCI-sponsored clinical trials available for your diagnosis. This service is completely free of charge.

However, the NCI generally does not provide information about clinical trials that it does not sponsor, and that includes many clinical trials sponsored by pharmaceutical companies. For trials sponsored by pharmaceutical companies, your best bet is the CenterWatch Clinical Trials Listing Service, which is described in the next section.

The Internet

If you're searching for cancer clinical trials yourself, and you've decided not to use the Cancer Information Service or hire a professional researcher (see "Research services," later in this chapter), you'll find a treasure trove of information on the Internet. The problem with treasure troves, however, is distinguishing items that are truly golden from those that are merely gold plated. This is a challenge not only for amateur Internet surfers, but also for highly experienced professional researchers as well. Pam Geyer of MEDcetera, Inc., observes:

> It's very difficult to get good quality information off the Internet because you have to know the difference between what is a commercial web site and what is peer-reviewed information. Even when I'm on the Internet, I have to be careful that I'm not pulling down biased, commercial information.

What follows is a collection of some sites on the World Wide Web and other segments of the Internet where you can find information on cancer clinical trials. Web sites spring up, change their character, and disappear continually, so this collection is almost certainly not exhaustive.

PDQ

The premier web page for finding clinical trials is the NCI's PDQ (Physician's Data Query) site. Originally intended for use only by medical professionals, PDQ is now designed to be so simple to use that practically anyone can zero in on the best clinical trials for specific cancers.

Located at *http://cancertrials.nci.nih.gov/*, PDQ is an easily searchable registry of more than 1,500 clinical trials for cancer. These include trials conducted by NCI-sponsored researchers, the pharmaceutical industry, and some international groups. The search form allows you to pick out all the trials for a certain type of cancer, and if that search returns too many "hits," you can further limit the search to trials of only certain types of treatments or trials of a certain phase. Furthermore, you can use PDQ to find all the trials on a specific drug, or those that are being conducted in a particular state. One of the nicest features of the search form is that you can ask it to show you only the newest trials, the ones that have been added within the last month. This is especially useful if your search for an appropriate clinical trial is an ongoing one.

On one recent autumn morning, PDQ turned up four clinical trials related to adrenocortical cancer. Initially, PDQ will give you only the names of the trials, but if you click in the boxes next to the names and then click the Display button, you'll get brief lay-language summaries of each of the trials. Those summaries include the rationale, purpose, and abbreviated eligibility requirements for the trial. There will also be a short description of the treatment, and you'll find the name, institution, and phone number of the principal investigator. If the trial is being conducted at more than one institution, you'll get the names and phone numbers of the principal investigators at all of those institutions. One of the clinical trials for adrenocortical cancer, for example, is a multicenter trial being conducted at no fewer than 66 institutions all around the country. Every one is listed. You should use your printer to get a hard copy of the summary of any interesting trial.

A nice feature of these summaries is that all potentially unfamiliar terms are hotlinked to their definitions. One of the other trials for adrenocortical cancer, for example, provides hotlinks that define the terms chemotherapy, Phase II trial, combination chemotherapy, doxorubicin, vincristine, etoposide, mitotane, measurable disease, and continuous infusion. But it's the final hotlink in each summary that's the most important. That one takes you to the health professional abstract of the trial.

The health professional abstract contains far more detail about the trial than does the summary. In particular, you'll learn about all the specific inclusion and exclusion criteria, such as what lab results will qualify you for—or disqualify you from—the study. Be sure to get a hard copy of the health professional abstract as well, even if you can't understand every word. Your physician will be happy to have this additional information.

As mentioned earlier in the section on the National Cancer Institute, you don't need Internet access to get information from PDQ. A telephone call to (800) 4-CANCER will get you to a researcher who will conduct a customized search of PDQ for free and will mail you the results.

Although PDQ is the best place to find clinical trials, even the NCI admits that it's not comprehensive. It's updated only once a month, and it also might not include every single trial sponsored by pharmaceutical companies. For that reason, your search shouldn't end with PDQ.

CenterWatch

The next place to search is the CenterWatch Clinical Trials Listing Service (*http://www.centerwatch.com*), which contains a searchable database of 7,500 current clinical trials in all areas of medicine, including cancer. Sponsored by CenterWatch, Inc., a Boston-based company that publishes several books, newsletters, and other services for the clinical trial industry, the Listing Service tends to have excellent coverage of pharmaceutical company-sponsored trials, but it's not nearly as comprehensive as PDQ. On the same day that PDQ turned up four trials on adrenal cancer, CenterWatch turned up none, and where PDQ found 36 trials for bladder cancer, CenterWatch found only 10. Several of those 10 were apparently not on the PDQ list, however, illustrating the value of searching both sites. Nancy Oster confirms this: "CenterWatch doesn't have all the trials that are on the NCI site, and vice versa. There is no central clearinghouse."

One problem with the CenterWatch trial listings is that they are far shorter and less detailed than the PDQ listings. Instead of providing the specifics of the treatment under study, many CenterWatch listings will only mention that it's a study of "an investigational treatment." For more information, you need to fill out a form on the web page and submit it, after which you'll be sent additional information in email.

The CenterWatch web site also has several other services of interest to people searching for cancer clinical trials. If you sign up for its Patient Notification Service, you'll get an email whenever a new clinical trial is listed in the areas you specify. There's also a link to a comprehensive listing of new drugs recently approved by the FDA. And under the heading of Professional Resources, CenterWatch will give you detailed profiles of research institutions, pharmaceutical companies, and contract research organizations that conduct clinical trials.

Medline

Although PDQ and CenterWatch are the best places to find lists of clinical trials, the National Library of Medicine (NLM) maintains a database called Medline that is by far the best place to search the medical literature for detailed information about cancer research and particular treatments. Medline has indexed virtually every article that has appeared in every scientific and medical journal, in English and other languages, since 1966. Until fairly recently, however, using Medline was fairly complex. It involved setting up a payment account, having your computer dial a special number to connect directly to the NLM's computers, and using an arcane set of computer commands to search the database.

Now, the process is much easier. Medline is available for free through several Internet sites, and searching the database has become simpler. Using Medline is still a bit tricky, however, and then there's the question of how to interpret what you find.

There are few if any lay-language summaries on Medline. What you'll get are dense, jargon-filled abstracts of highly technical articles from English and foreign-language scientific and medical literature. But if you can understand this information—or if you can find someone to explain it to you—it will be an invaluable aid in deciding among various treatment options and clinical trials.

There are two especially good ways of accessing Medline on the Internet. You'll find Internet Grateful Med at *http://igm.nlm.nih.gov/*, and you'll find PubMed at *http://www4.ncbi.nlm.nih.gov/PubMed/*. PubMed is simpler to use and more straightforward, but Grateful Med is more flexible and powerful.

One limitation of Medline is that it won't give you the full text of the article. At the most, you'll get an abstract—a single (sometimes lengthy) paragraph briefly describing the study and its results. If you want to read the full article, in most cases you'll have to find it in a medical library.

When downloading the results of a Medline search, be sure to request those abstracts. Otherwise, you'll find yourself trying to decide whether an article is important on the basis of its title alone. The titles of scientific papers are often relatively uninformative and densely filled with jargon. Even though abstracts are themselves frequently difficult to decode, you have a better chance of figuring things out by using abstracts than the title alone.

Cancer center web sites

If you live near a major cancer center, it's worthwhile visiting its web site in search of clinical trials. Some cancer centers make it easy to find clinical trials. The M.D. Anderson Cancer Center in Houston, Texas, for example, has a link to all its clinical trials right on its main page (*http://www.mdanderson.org/*). Other cancer centers, either intentionally or through poor organization, make it difficult to find their clinical trials. Nancy Oster relates an experience she had:

> *I read in the media that there was a trial at [a well-known cancer hospital]. So I went to their web site to try to find it, and that was a nightmare. It actually is on their web site, but you really, really have to search. Even knowing what I was searching for, even knowing what it was called and what was involved, I had a real hard time finding it. I finally found the department that was doing it, and then I found the description of the trial. And sometimes, there's this caginess about letting people know about trials. I don't quite understand what the purpose of that is. When I called [the cancer hospital]—because I wanted to get a listing of all their trials for our Breast Cancer Resource Center—the woman said, "We prefer to have people call us and go through a preliminary interview before we identify which trials are available to them," which felt really funny to me. I don't understand why the information is being kept behind closed doors.*

News release collections

When an institution starts a clinical trial, it's usually eager to recruit patients. Often, one of the first things it does is distribute a news release, describing the clinical trial in lay language. In the days before the Internet, it would mail these news releases to local and national reporters to make it easy for them to write articles about the trials.

Institutions still put news releases in the US mail, but increasingly, they're putting them online as well. Several services contain large collections of news releases from hundreds of institutions. Some of these services maintain searchable archives of news releases going back several years. This provides a wonderful opportunity for the general public because anyone can get information about new clinical trials directly from the source, without waiting for articles to appear through the filter of the news media.

The oldest of these services is PR Newswire (*http://www.prnewswire.com/*), which has been transmitting news releases to news rooms via teletype since 1954. Although PR Newswire's web site contains many current news releases, and you can search for any term in those releases, you'll only be able to find material released within the last week. Additionally, although PR Newswire tends to be quite a good source for business news, it's not as good a source for health and medical news. But because many pharmaceutical companies like to announce the start of new clinical trials to the investment community, frequent visits to PR Newswire might pay off in early warnings of interesting trials. You can also find material from PR Newswire using the Excite Newstracker service (described in the next section).

Two other services compile and index news releases primarily from academic institutions, including most major medical centers. They are EurekAlert (*http://www.eurekalert.org/*), which is run by the American Association for the Advancement of Science, and Newswise (*http://www.newswise.com/*), which is run by science writer Roger Johnson. Both sites have extensive archives of news releases going back several years, and both add new releases continually. Although many institutions place their releases in both EurekAlert and Newswise, some use only one or the other, so it's worthwhile checking both.

Excite Newstracker

The World Wide Web provides several means of searching news articles on any given topic, and one of the best is Excite's Newstracker service (*http://nt.excite.com/*). Excite continually indexes all the articles from more than 300 publications with contents on the Web, including major newspapers such as *The New York Times* and the *Washington Post* and important sources of medical information such as the *New England Journal of Medicine* and the *UC Berkeley*

Wellness Letter. It even indexes some news release sites, including EurekAlert and PR Newswire (but not Newswise).

Newstracker will let you set up "custom topics" so you can run the same search day after day or week after week. This is an excellent way of keeping up with the latest news about clinical trials for your cancer. When setting up a custom topic, be specific, but not too specific, about what you're looking for. When you're searching the popular press, you'll want to search for "adrenal cancer." Simply looking for "cancer" or "clinical trials" will give you too much irrelevant information, and a highly specific search term such as "inoperable stage III adrenocortical carcinoma" is likely to return nothing at all.

Because Newstracker is updated continually, whereas services such as PDQ are only updated monthly, you may find a clinical trial with Newstracker before it's listed in the official NCI site.

Email discussion lists and Usenet newsgroups

Another way to find information about cancer clinical trials and other treatments on the Internet is to look to patient support groups. There are generally two types of patient support groups on the Internet: those based on email and those based on Usenet newsgroups.

By far, the best collection of email discussion groups on cancer is maintained by ACOR, the Association of Cancer Online Resources, at *http://www.medinfo.org/*. Click on Join a List, and you'll be presented with the names and brief descriptions of 80 mailing lists on all types and aspects of cancer, ranging from the Aplastic Anemia and Myleodysplastic Syndrome list to the Waldenstrom Macroglobulenemia list. If you're interested in information that's not related to a specific type of cancer, you can also subscribe to CANCER-L for general discussions. You might want to start by searching the past messages to the lists, which are fully archived. All of this is completely free.

Once you subscribe to the list, your email box will fill with impassioned and informative messages on every aspect of your illness, contributed by people who are fighting these illnesses, their families, and healthcare providers. There will be discussions of all the various treatment options and clinical trials, and chances are that another subscriber will be participating in any trial you might be considering. Once you join an email discussion list, posting questions or comments of your own is as easy as sending an email message.

Some lists are so busy, and some topics generate so much discussion, that it's not unusual for an email discussion list to generate more than 100 messages each day. To avoid having all these messages overflow your mail box, subscribe to the digest version of the list. (You'll find instructions on how to do this on the ACOR site.) A digest subscription will give you a single message each day that contains the full text of all the previous day's individual messages.

You can also find support groups on Usenet, a collection of more than 20,000 newsgroups on every conceivable subject. Five of those groups will interest people with cancer:

- alt.support.cancer
- alt.support.cancer.breast
- alt.support.cancer.prostate
- alt.support.cancer.testicular
- sci.med.diseases.cancer

Providing full instructions for participating in Usenet newsgroups is beyond the scope of this book; you can learn to use newsgroups by using news reader software that's often included in full-featured Internet browsers such as Netscape Communicator and Microsoft

Internet Explorer. You can also access Usenet newsgroups through a web site called Deja News, *http://www.dejanews.com/*.

It is important to remember several things about any patient support group, whether it's an email discussion list or a Usenet newsgroup. One is that you should take everything that's said in these groups with a large grain of salt. Although many participants are well meaning and well informed, some are misinformed, others have axes to grind, and a few are actively malevolent. Double check everything.

Occasionally, long arguments called flame wars break out in these groups. Some of these flame wars descend into insults and personal attacks. On other occasions, people with, shall we say, idiosyncratic ideas, shout loudly to be heard. The newsgroups alt.support.cancer and sci.med.diseases.cancer are frequently host to the offensive and obsessive rants of individuals who are convinced that leukemia is not a real disease, but instead is an evil conspiracy of doctors and pharmaceutical companies to extort money from deluded patients. Other participants are snake-oil salesmen, whose shameful *modus operandi* is to peddle their quack remedies to vulnerable and desperate people.

Enter these support groups equipped with healthy skepticism and a good suit of flame-proof armor, or you may find that they do more harm than good. Used properly, they can provide not only valuable information, but also a community of like-minded individuals who are going through what you're going through.

Gary Schine offers his take on support groups:

> *As far as I'm concerned, a lot of support groups put a great deal of emphasis on talking about illness but almost downplay doing anything practical, like getting rid of it. A support group is an adjunct to the important concern: finding the best way to treat your illness.*

WebMD

Numerous other health and medical web sites are springing up, many of which contain information about cancer and clinical trials. It isn't possible to list them all here, but one of the most interesting is WebMD (*http://my.webmd.com/*). WebMD is a collection of communities of people with serious health concerns. As this is being written, it has only three cancer communities—for breast cancer, ovarian cancer, and prostate cancer—but according to Paul Sonnenschein, WebMD's senior vice president, WebMD plans to start several other cancer communities in the near future, including ones for cervical cancer, endometrial cancer, and colorectal cancer. Members of the community can discuss issues related to their illness in message boards similar to Usenet newsgroups, and they can also interact in real time in chat rooms. WebMD frequently stages discussions with scientific and medical experts that are open to all members. Because these message boards and discussions are moderated, flame wars and off-topic posts are much less of a problem than they are in Usenet newsgroups or email discussion lists.

The nicest thing about WebMD is that it will contact you if a pharmaceutical company retains them to recruit patients for a clinical trial for which you may qualify. It does this by having you answer a detailed medical questionnaire when you sign up. You needn't worry about divulging too much private information, however; you never have to give your real name or any other identifying information aside from a nickname and your email address. And if you're worried about giving out your regular email address, you can always sign up for a free email address from a service such as Hotmail (*http://www.hotmail.com/*), Mailexcite (*http://www.mailexcite.com/*), or Yahoo Mail (*http://mail.yahoo.com/*).

Paul Sonnenschein talks about WebMD:

> *We create disease-specific web sites that are focused around chronic and serious conditions like breast cancer. And we then work with pharmaceutical and medical device companies in pro-*

viding anonymous access to these patients for market research, for
patient education programs, and also for doing trial recruitment.
When we sign up a patient for our site, we don't ask for their
name, address, or Social Security number. All we do is ask them to
fill out a detailed medical profile, and we ask them to give us their
email address and to choose a nickname and a password. And we
never divulge that nickname, email address, or password to any
outside company without the express consent of the patient.
Because we gather information in detail about someone's medical
condition, their treatment path, and so on, we can target solicita-
tions to patients who are presenting certain kinds of symptoms or
who have certain kinds of side effects from other treatments.
Patients are not inundated with solicitations. They are approached
only when it makes sense.

The news media

Your local newspaper is another source of information about clinical trials, but the information you find there will be far from
comprehensive, and you might find yourself chasing down many
blind alleys. Occasionally, you'll see news articles in which the
reporter describes the latest exciting "breakthrough" in cancer
research. Unfortunately, many such articles describe research that's
been performed only in test tubes or on animals. Although some of
this research might sound promising, the history of the War on
Cancer is replete with treatments that killed cancer cells in the test
tube or even cured cancer in mice but were ineffective—or had
unacceptable toxicity—in humans.

If you were to contact the researchers mentioned in these articles,
as many people with cancer do, you'll often find that human clinical trials are many months or years away. Frequently, the scientists
quoted in these articles are basic researchers who are not involved
in clinical trials at all. Such scientists are typically inundated with
calls from desperate cancer patients and their families soon after
articles describing their research appear in the popular press, but

they can usually offer no encouragement or even information about when clinical trials might begin.

When you read an article on a potential cancer advance, be sure to look closely for information about whether human clinical trials are planned and, if so, when they will start and where they will be conducted. In the absence of those details, chasing those leads will usually prove fruitless and frustrating.

Rather than pin your hopes on news articles describing laboratory advances, look for articles that specifically mention clinical trials. When a medical institution begins a clinical trial, it's often eager to recruit patients, and the institution's public relations people will issue a news release that they mail to local reporters. These reporters will sometimes write articles about the trial, but unless the trial is a large one that is national in scope, the articles will be short, and they'll be buried in the back pages of the paper or possibly in the paper's health or lifestyles section. It's worthwhile keeping an eye out for these articles.

You can also gain direct access to news releases announcing clinical trials by using the EurekAlert, Newswise, or Newstracker services described previously.

Sometimes, institutions running clinical trials will purchase newspaper advertisements. It's hard to find these ads unless you know where to look, and they tend to appear in different places in different newspapers. In some papers, you'll find ads for clinical trials in the classified section, under General Announcements. In other papers, institutions advertising clinical trials will purchase display ads. These tend to appear in the health or lifestyles section. And occasionally, you'll hear ads for clinical trials on the radio, more frequently on talk radio than on music stations. On rare occasions, you might even see an ad for a clinical trial on television.

The problem with using the news media to find cancer clinical trials is that the media cover clinical trials only haphazardly.

Many—probably most—trials are never mentioned in the news media at all, not before, not during, and not after they're conducted. For that reason, poring over piles of newspapers has little place in an organized strategy for finding clinical trials. But it's worth keeping an eye on the media just the same.

Libraries

Your local library—even if it's a community library—is probably an excellent source of basic information about your cancer. Once you've gleaned what you can from the library's own reference works, check out the databases. Many libraries subscribe to a CD-ROM-based system called InfoTrac that contains health-based information from 150 medical journals; 500 pamphlets; 2,500 general-interest publications; and 5 popular medical reference books. InfoTrac is updated monthly and its index goes back three years.

More local libraries now provide terminals connected to the Internet. Through those terminals, you'll be able to get to all the sites mentioned in the Internet section earlier in this chapter. The one possible exception to this is libraries that have installed software intended to prevent people from getting to "objectionable" sites, such as those that are sexually oriented. Some of that software is so poorly written that it'll block you from visiting sites related to breast cancer! If that happens, complain to the librarian. It might be possible to temporarily remove the block.

With the exception of information available through their Internet terminals, however, most local libraries lack detailed medical information and information directly related to clinical trials. For that, you'll need to find a medical library. There's a medical library in nearly every hospital, although some are not open to the public. Some medical libraries are very limited, with little more than a selection of recent journals. Others, typically found in major academic medical centers, are large and comprehensive, with miles of shelves holding thousands of books. These libraries also maintain archives of hundreds or thousands of medical journals going back many decades. Some of these libraries have Internet connections available for public use and direct connections to Medline and other database services. Best of all, some medical libraries have highly experienced medical librarians, who will sometimes conduct searches for a modest fee. According to Nancy Oster:

> *Some medical libraries will do a search on a topic for $20 or $25. They're also really good at getting you started, giving you guidance in the right direction.*

Research services

For a more thorough search, at a somewhat higher fee, you might want to consider hiring a research service. (All services mentioned in this section are listed in Appendix A, *Resources*.) At a cost of no more than a few hundred dollars, you can hire an experienced researcher to prepare a detailed report that will include the latest medical research about your kind of cancer, along with lists of all available clinical trials. Nancy Oster notes:

> *When you're in a crisis situation and you don't really have the time to learn all this stuff and to do it efficiently, then it seems as if it does make sense to get that jump start. Then you can take off from there and do some research on your own as well. It's not an all-or-nothing thing.*

Research services are great for people who have little experience using the Internet. It's far quicker—and a great deal less expensive—to hire someone to do research for you than to assemble the necessary equipment and teach yourself how to do it on your own. Even if you're experienced in using computers, you might find value in using professional researchers, especially if you have no particular expertise in cancer research and clinical trials. Gary Schine of Schine On-Line Services says:

> *Oftentimes I'll hear something like, "Yes, I know how to use the Internet. In fact, I'm a computer programmer, and I've been at it*

for 30 years. But it's easier to pay you 200 bucks than to learn how to do it myself."

Gary Schine gained his expertise in researching cancer clinical trials the hard way. Diagnosed in 1991 at the age of 38 with hairy-cell leukemia, Schine refused to accept that his only hope was major surgery—the removal of his spleen—followed by chemotherapy. Schine knew that at best, these treatments would delay his death. He wanted a cure, so he set out to find it. Find it he did, in a Phase II clinical trial of a new chemotherapy agent called 2-chlorodeoxyadenosine (2-CDA). The FDA approved 2-CDA in 1993, and eight years following his treatment, Schine remains in full remission with no evidence of disease.

Shortly after his recovery, Schine started Schine On-Line Services. Through this company, he provides lengthy and detailed research reports on any illness, although he specializes in cancer. This report will range from 80 to 200 pages in length. It currently costs $195, and can be sent to you in one or two business days. It includes:

- An overview of your illness written for the layperson.

- A more technical overview of your illness.

- A list of current clinical trials for your illness with all important details, including names, addresses, and phone numbers for the person and organization leading each clinical trial as well as the names of all doctors and institutions near you who are authorized to administer those trials.

- The latest treatment-related developments for your illness from more than 3,000 English and foreign-language medical and scientific journals.

- Information on alternative and non-traditional approaches to your illness.

- A list of medical libraries in your area for follow-up research.

Pam Geyer runs a similar service called MEDcetera. For $135 plus shipping, she'll provide a nicely bound 30- to 50-page report on your illness, plus a lengthy list of available clinical trials, and she generally ships these reports within 24 hours.

Another professional research service is The Health Resource, which will provide a report within four to five working days for $275 to $375.

These services are listed as samples only, and their description here should not be taken to imply endorsement. You can find additional research services by searching for "consumer health research" at Yahoo (*http://www.yahoo.com/*).

Once you've found candidate trials

Once you've developed a list of trials that might be appropriate for your situation, the difficult problem of evaluating them begins. You might be able to cross some off the list by closely perusing the eligibility requirements; if the study excludes people who have had previous chemotherapy, and you've had chemotherapy, it would be a waste of your time—and the investigator's—to call for more information.

You might be able to reject other trials because they don't seem promising on the basis of your other research as they would require an unacceptable amount of travel, or the study won't be getting underway for six months. Bear in mind that some of these problems might not be insurmountable. If travel is a problem, your local oncologist might be able to administer some of the treatments, for example.

Once you've eliminated the trials that aren't appropriate, you or your doctor should start phoning the investigators running the remaining trials. Don't be shy about phoning; patient recruitment is one of the most difficult aspects of running a clinical trial, and most investigators or members of their staffs are delighted to speak with patients or their families. Often you'll be referred to a research nurse or a physician assistant who is conducting the preliminary screening. He'll ask you a series of questions to determine whether you qualify for the trial. If it seems that you do, he'll most likely make an appointment for an examination.

Lydia Cunningham Rising offers this advice for contacting the researcher:

> Just call the researcher yourself. You don't have to be referred by your doctor. You can call up anybody, and most of them will talk to you. Here's a trick: if you reach a secretary who asks to take a message, don't leave one, since the researcher doesn't know your name and may not call you back. Make an excuse—say that you'll be away from your phone or something—and ask, "When would be a good time for me to call him?" Invariably they will say, "The doctor will be in his office around 3 p.m. on Friday."

You'll be asked to bring a good deal in the way of medical records with you to the initial examination. Your physician might also be asked to write a summary of your case. It is almost always the patient's responsibility to gather this material and get it to the people running the clinical trial. You or a family member might have to pester your physician or your medical plan until they come through with the necessary material.

More advice from Lydia Cunningham Rising:

> Even if the doctor's an S.O.B., most of the stuff the researcher needs is not in the doctor's possession. If you had blood tests or a CT scan, there's a copy at the hospital. You just ignore the doctor and get whatever you can from other sources. You may have to bug the hospital. I once had to ask a hospital for a CT scan, and based on their response, you'd think that copying a CT scan involved a team of monks in the back room using calligraphy! But it turns out that they just stick it into a big machine and the copy

comes right out. It's amazing the trouble they will give you over nothing. Once they've copied it, you may want to make sure they don't send it by donkey mail. I would offer to have it Federal Expressed.

For detailed help in deciding whether to participate in an individual clinical trial, see Chapter 7, *Evaluating a Clinical Trial.*

CHAPTER FIVE

Special Types of Trials

WHEN WE THINK OF EXPERIMENTAL cancer treatments, we tend to think of drugs intended to make the disease disappear. These treatments go through the familiar Phase I, Phase II, Phase III sequence described in Chapter 2, *The Structure of Clinical Trials*. But not all cancer research is aimed squarely at making an individual's disease disappear, and there are some exceptions to the typical sequence.

This chapter discusses trials of preventive and adjuvant therapies, trials of supportive therapies, and trials for new surgical techniques and new medical devices. The chapter concludes with a discussion of genetic trials, which might not help individual participants, but which might ultimately lead to a true understanding—and, we hope, a true cure—for cancer.

Adjuvant therapy and prevention trials

Some clinical trials are intended to test ways to prevent the appearance or reappearance of cancer in people who are at risk. Adjuvant trials are for people who have had cancer that has been successfully treated by surgery, radiation therapy, chemotherapy, or other means. Medication is then given as an adjuvant—literally, "an assistant"—in the hope of preventing a recurrence of the cancer.

Don Sterner relates his experience:

> *I was still in the hospital recovering from surgery. The doctor in the hematological section came over several times and explained*

that my tumor had been removed completely with clear margins,
but they wanted to do chemotherapy as a precautionary measure
because a lot of these tumors spread.

Dr. Ephraim Resnik is a gynecological oncologist at St. Louis University School of Medicine. He explains adjuvant treatment this way:

When you have somebody with a measurable disease and you're
treating them with chemotherapy, you're basically looking for a
response. You're watching the size of the lesion shrink, remain the
same, or (sometimes, unfortunately) grow. With an adjuvant trial,
the major difference from a research standpoint is that you have
different end points. You don't have measurable disease, something
you can feel or see on the x-ray. There, the end point is time to
recurrence of the disease and overall survival.

Prevention trials are similar to adjuvant-therapy trials in that the investigators are looking for an increase in survival time or an increase in the time to the appearance of the disease. These end points tend to be difficult to measure statistically because many people who are at risk will never develop cancer even without the experimental intervention. For that reason, investigators must enroll thousands of people to have any hope of getting a statistically significant result.

Prevention trials are almost always randomized (except in the earliest phases), and many are double-blind; neither the investigators nor the participants know who is getting the study medication.

Tamoxifen is a recent example of a drug proven in clinical trials to be a valuable adjuvant therapy for some women with breast cancer. More recently, the FDA has approved tamoxifen for use as a risk-reduction therapy. According to medical oncologist Abigail A. Silvers:

There have been adjuvant trials with tamoxifen. That gave us
the idea that it might be used as a preventive as well. Women who

had one breast cancer and were felt to be at risk to get a recur-
rence of that disease were given tamoxifen. And it was found that
tamoxifen lowered the risk of recurrence, and it also lowered the
risk of getting cancer in the opposite breast. If it can prevent it in
the opposite breast of women who'd already had breast cancer,
why not try it in women who were at above average risk for breast
cancer? Prevention is where we want to go. It would be much bet-
ter for people to be healthy and never develop a disease.

Dr. Silvers, who participated as a principal investigator at Bryn Mawr Hospital (Bryn Mawr, Pennsylvania) in the recent nationwide Breast Cancer Prevention Trial, notes that such trials differ in a number of respects from therapeutic trials. For one thing, the researchers must follow trial participants for a much longer period of time:

We don't know how much time it takes for diseases to develop,
and we also don't know how long a particular drug will work after
you stop it. For the tamoxifen study, we followed the women for
five years while on the drug and will continue to follow them for at
least two years after they stop the medication.

Dr. Resnik, who was an investigator in the same trial at his institution, agrees: "A prevention trial is a bigger commitment for physicians, for institutions, and for the patients."

Prevention trials also have significant differences from treatment trials in the way participants are recruited and informed consent is conducted. Dr. Silvers explains:

Recruitment for prevention trials is much harder because basi-
cally these are healthy people, and you're probably going to give
them some side effects from whatever preventive measures you're
testing. So it's a real weighing of risks and of your degree of altru-
ism if you're a candidate.

Healthy women going into a prevention trial are just not going
to put up with side effects that somebody going into a treatment

trial will put up with. It's often a lengthier consent form for a prevention trial. In the breast cancer tamoxifen trial, it was sixteen
pages long, versus six pages in one for a treatment trial. It went
into great detail on the possible side effects.

Dr. Resnik points out:

> When you're dealing with an essentially healthy person, you
> have to be very thorough to make sure that the person understands
> a variety of different big and little untoward events that can hap-
> pen during the trial.

Dr. Resnik also notes that some insurance companies have a different attitude about prevention trials than about therapeutic trials.
(For more information about insurance coverage of clinical trials,
see Chapter 9, *Financial Issues*.)

> Insurance companies are less likely to cover prevention trials
> because the benefit there is not clearly defined. In one study I was
> involved in, there were issues of endometrial sampling and of
> doing ultrasound on patients. Insurance companies were willing to
> pay for it in about half of the patients that I personally was
> involved with. The other half had to pay out of pocket.

Trials of supportive therapies

Not every cancer clinical trial is aimed squarely at finding a cure for
the disease. Many clinical trials are intended to find treatments to
alleviate some of the consequences of cancer or the side effects of
some cancer treatments. These are generally referred to as supportive therapies.

Many chemotherapeutic regimens cause nausea, for example. If
that's a problem for you, and none of the standard antiemetic (antinausea) medications work well enough, you might want to look for
a clinical trial.

Pain is an unfortunate consequence of many types of cancer. If none of the standard analgesics are working well for you, you might be able to find a clinical trial for new analgesics.

There are many other examples. A recent search of the NCI's PDQ database yielded a list of 105 trials of supportive therapies. This wide-ranging list includes a trial of a smoking-cessation program for early stage cancer patients, a trial of a drug intended to prevent dry-mouth syndrome in patients receiving radiation therapy for head and neck cancers, and a trial of a drug for treating the heart damage that's a possible side effect of a chemotherapy regimes using anthracycline for childhood cancers.

Even if you're satisfied with your current cancer treatment, it's worth taking a look at the list of supportive therapy trials to see whether there's a trial involving one of the symptoms at the periphery of your disease. Such a trial could improve your quality of life during treatment.

Trials of new surgical techniques

Although surgery sometimes seems more of an art than a science, even surgical techniques must be proven to work. Clinical trials for new surgical techniques have certain differences from trials for other types of treatments. The most obvious difference is that there are really no Phase I surgical clinical trials because there's clearly no need to find the right dose of surgery. It is important, however, to define the extent and the timing of surgery in the context of all of a patient's treatment when designing a surgical trial.

Dr. David Jablons, a thoracic surgeon, says of surgical trials:

> There's no dose escalation in a surgical trial. A new surgical technique either makes a difference or it doesn't. The early phase data goes very fast. If you don't get good results, or you get dramatically better results with this technique than previous techniques, it rapidly becomes clear. Then you may do a head-to-head Phase III randomized trial.

Occasionally it can be a challenge to interpret the results of a surgical clinical trial. For one thing, there's no way to conduct single- or double-blind studies. Both the patient and the surgeon will always know which type of surgery has been performed, the surgeon because he was there and the patient because of consent forms and telltale scars. In addition, as Dr. Jablons explains, with different surgeons performing the operations, there's also the question of whether different surgeons are performing the exact same operation:

> *The issue there is operator variance. It's one thing if you have ten centers running a drug trial, and they all get one set of pills from a central warehouse. But if you have ten different centers and ten different thoracic surgeons, they may each do the operation a little differently. They all do it the same general way, but there are some style-point variations.*

One of the hot areas of surgical innovation these days involves minimally invasive surgery. Instead of making a large incision and opening the entire chest cavity—to remove a tumor, for example— surgeons are learning how to accomplish the same result by making several tiny incisions through which they insert their surgical instruments, including a thoracascope—a device that lets the surgeons see what they're doing through an eyepiece or on a video screen.

Patients tend to prefer minimally invasive surgery because their surgical wounds heal much faster than they would have otherwise and they can spend less time in the hospital. But some surgeons remain skeptical about this technique, says Dr. Jablons, because it makes it harder for the surgeon to see what's going on and to do things such as stitch blood vessels. A single tiny stitch that's placed in a slightly suboptimal spot can lead to disaster a few weeks or months later. These sort of risks should be clearly explained to you if you're considering a surgical clinical trial, and if they're not, you should be sure to ask about them.

Medical device trials

Medical devices go through a somewhat different approval process than do drugs or other types of treatments. (See Chapter 8 *Administration of Clinical Trials*, for a description of a drug's route to approval.) As in clinical trials of new surgical techniques, there's really no need to conduct Phase I dose escalation studies, for example.

In fact, not all new medical devices have to go through clinical trials. For the purposes of regulation, the FDA divides medical devices into three classes:

- **Class I.** These devices present the least risk and are subject to the fewest controls. They include bandages and gauze. Clinical trials are rarely required for Class I devices.

- **Class II.** These devices carry intermediate risk and are subject to moderate controls. They often contain some technological component, but if the manufacturer can show that its new device uses technology that has been used successfully for quite some time, clinical trials might not be required.

- **Class III.** These devices are considered to carry the most risk. They include devices using new technology as well as devices that have critical safety implications, such as pacemakers or respirators. Clinical trials will almost always be required for new Class III devices.

A good example of a medical device that's in clinical trials as this is being written is the Biofield Diagnostic System, which is intended to be a less invasive way of diagnosing breast cancer than the biopsy that follows a suspicious mammogram. The device is being manufactured by the Biofield Corporation of Roswell, Georgia. Robert M. Johnson, Biofield's Chief Operating Officer explains:

> *If you look at the way breast cancer is diagnosed today, it's a time-consuming, laborious process that fills a woman with apprehension. It would be nice if before all of that began, you could do a*

direct test, much like an EKG, and hopefully prevent a lot of these women from ever beginning the testing milieu.

The test actually is much like the common electrocardiogram used to diagnose heart ailments. In the case of the Biofield Diagnostic System, a number of electrodes are attached with adhesive to the outside of the breast, surrounding the suspicious lump. A few minutes of electrical readings are taken, and then the electrodes are removed.

The theory behind the device is that the electrical properties of a malignant tumor will differ from normal tissue. If this theory proves valid in clinical trials, more people may be able to avoid biopsies, many of which prove unnecessary because mammography has a high number of "false positives"—suspicious shadows on the x-ray that turn out to be nothing.

For the clinical trials, which are being conducted at a number of sites in the US and Europe, investigators are recruiting women who are headed for biopsies as a result of a suspicious mammogram.

Mr. Johnson describes what participants are told about the trial:

They're all told that the information cannot be used to treat them, that it will be used to help the development of the device, which, in the long run, may prove to be beneficial to other patients if and when the device is commercialized.

In fact, the women are never even informed of their test results, so they can't change their minds about the biopsy if the test seems to show that they don't have a malignancy. This is because the investigators need to compare results from the new device to results from the biopsy as a means of proving whether the device actually works.

This means that, for this device at least, there is no direct benefit whatsoever to a woman participating in this trial, other than the personal satisfaction of knowing that she has helped advance medical science. On the other hand, participating in this trial takes only a short amount of time, and the risk is very small. In fact, the worst thing that seems to happen is that some women have a mild, transient reaction to the adhesive used to attach the electrode to the skin.

When considering a medical-device trial, be sure you're clear about whether you can expect any direct benefit from your participation. Be sure you know also how much inconvenience is involved and whether you're likely to experience any pain or discomfort.

Genetic trials

One of the most exciting and productive areas of basic cancer research involves looking for genetic markers or genes that predispose one to or directly cause certain types of cancer. This book is not the place for a detailed discussion of this field of research. Suffice it to say, however, that to discover a gene that causes cancer would be to find a single short stretch of DNA along one of your 46 chromosomes that, when activated, directly leads to cells becoming cancerous. Sometimes a certain gene greatly increases the chance that an individual will get cancer, although it doesn't cause the disease by itself. Perhaps additional, environmental factors are necessary to cause the disease to appear. Such a gene is said to predispose someone to get cancer.

A genetic marker, on the other hand, would be a short, recognizable stretch of DNA that appears in many people who get a certain type of cancer and does not appear in close relatives who don't get the disease. A genetic marker neither causes cancer nor predisposes one toward cancer; instead, its location on the chromosome is most likely very close to an as yet undiscovered gene that is somehow involved in the cancer.

The way researchers find cancer genes and genetic markers is to collect blood or tissue samples from people with cancer and their close relatives. Detailed and laborious analysis of the DNA in these cells—which sometimes takes years to perform—occasionally reveals cancer markers and cancer genes.

A recent search of NCI's PDQ database yielded a list of nine genetic trials for various types of cancer. Some of the trials involve tissue collected only from people with cancer, and others involve tissue collected from blood relatives as well.

A few things are important to know about genetic studies. First of all, it's extremely unlikely that you will receive any direct benefit if you choose to participate. In fact, you will most likely never learn the results of the study or whether the sample you provided contained a genetic marker or a cancer gene. That also goes for any relatives of yours who might participate.

Second, you might be asked for a list of blood relatives, along with their addresses and phone numbers. The researchers will then contact your relatives and ask them to participate in the trial by giving blood or tissue samples. None of your relatives will be required to participate. Each of them will go through the same informed consent process that you will, and each of them is free to decline to be part of the trial. However, some of them might not approve of your giving their names to investigators. Even if they do participate, they might have to live with the anxiety of wondering whether they inherited a cancer gene, and as previously noted, they will most likely never learn the answer to that question.

On the other hand, participation in genetic trials generally takes only a short time and usually involves nothing more painful than providing a blood sample. No area of cancer research offers more promise for finding the ultimate causes and cures for cancer. Participation in a genetic study is one of the easiest, yet most significant, ways that someone with cancer can contribute to cancer research.

CHAPTER SIX

Choosing Possible Trials

THIS CHAPTER DISCUSSES a few general considerations for narrowing your choice of trials and then looks at unique considerations involved in clinical trials for children and for people with advanced cancer.

No easy answers

It would be nice if one could develop a highly definitive set of rules for choosing clinical trials. If we had these, we could print a chart in this book that would match your type and stage of cancer with the best kind of clinical trial: Do you have stage II sosablastoma? Simply find it on the chart and determine that you should look for a Phase III immunotherapy trial.

Unfortunately, its impossible to be so precise. There are many different kinds of cancer, and each person with cancer is unique. On top of that, there are about 1,500 cancer clinical trials underway in the US at any one time. Old trials are being completed and new ones are being added continually. Moreover, some experimental therapies that seem exciting and hopeful as this book is being written will be regarded as unfortunate blind alleys a year or two from now. Others that are now mere gleams in a researcher's eye will be in active clinical trials. Dr. David Jablons notes:

> *In a perfect world, it would be good if a lay person could have access to knowledge that would allow them to make the right, intelligent decision as to the best therapy for this disease. But it*

still unfortunately comes down to these huge gray areas about what the right treatment is or, in the lack of a known excellent treatment, how you make the right choice. You have to rely, I think, on people who are in the trenches who are doing this kind of work and can honestly say what their best hunch would be. The fundamental question would be: Okay Doc, what would you do if it were your mother or dad or brother or sister?

General considerations

Still, it's possible to make some general statements that could help you narrow your choices. In choosing a clinical trial, the most important thing you need is an honest assessment of your prognosis. Do you have a type of cancer that's easily cured by a simple surgical procedure? Do you have one for which current chemotherapy regimens are highly successful? Or do you have a type of cancer for which the five-year survival rate is under 10 percent? An unvarnished understanding of your prognosis provides the context for your decision making.

You also need to understand your own tolerance for risk and discomfort. Are you willing to try a highly experimental treatment that's likely to have severe side effects, or are you willing to take only small risks?

Lydia Cunningham Rising shares her opinion:

> *I tell people that if they have a poor prognosis, look for something that's really new. Just adjusting doses on chemotherapy isn't going to help you very much. You need to look for something different, something unique, rather than the same old same old. There are a lot of trials out there that are just diddling around with chemotherapy agents that don't have that much effect in the first place. On the other hand, if you had a cancer that responds to the chemotherapy decently well in the first place, go ahead and seek out these less interesting trials.*

Clinical trials for children

Children with cancer are far more likely to participate in clinical trials than their adult counterparts. According to the Pediatric Oncology Group, for example, 81 percent of children with cancer seen at their member institutions in 1997 were enrolled in clinical trials. Compare this to the NCI's estimate that less than 5 percent of adults with cancer participate in clinical trials. (See *Notes,* "Chapter 1: *Overview of Clinical Trials,*" for a discussion of this figure.)

Victor M. Santana, a pediatric oncologist/hematologist at St. Jude Children's Research Hospital in Memphis, Tennessee, believes that the ultimate reason for the greater participation among children is that childhood cancers, thank goodness, are relatively rare. As a consequence, there are few specialists in child oncology in private practice, and most of them are employed by major academic medical centers. Children with cancer are therefore likely to be seen in the very institutions—and by the very individuals—who administer the majority of clinical trials:

> *The development of clinical research protocol in children is no different than in adults. The methodology is no different. What is different is the diseases that are being treated. Most adult cancers are related somehow to environmental factors, to dietary factors, to styles of living. In contrast, most pediatric malignancies are embryologic disorders. It's not something they got from smoking or their diet. It's something that has gone wrong during embryonic development that makes this tissue become malignant.*

According to Nancy Keene, author of *Childhood Leukemia: A Guide for Families, Friends, & Caregivers*, 2nd Edition (O'Reilly & Associates, 1999):

> *Treatment of childhood ALL [acute lymphoblastic leukemia] is one of the major medical success stories of the last two decades. In the 1960s, patients with ALL usually lived only for a few months, but by the early 1990s, 70 percent of children receiving optimal treatment were cured.*

This gratifying result is the direct consequence of a high level of participation in cancer clinical trials by children. Despite the laudably high levels of participation, however, the level needs to be higher still. Until recently, pharmaceutical companies never tested the majority of drugs, cancer drugs included, on children. This might not be a problem if children could be regarded as miniature adults for the purposes of medical treatment. If that were the case, your doctor could simply scale down the dosage in proportion to the child's size.

Children, however, are not miniature adults. Because they have immature kidneys and livers, they metabolize drugs differently than adults. In addition, you have to consider the long-term consequences of the drug. When a physician gives a 50-year-old a highly toxic chemotherapy agent, she knows that even if the cancer goes into complete remission, the patient's life expectancy is probably no more than 20 or 30 years. But if she gives a 5-year-old the same chemotherapy agent, that patient may well have to live with the distant side effects of that drug for 80 years or more. Dr. Santana says:

> In performing research trials on pediatric oncology patients, we are very sensitive to the potential of long-term effects of therapy. For example, a concern is that you are treated and cured of one disease when you're 5 years old, but then 15 or 20 or 30 years later, you develop a second malignancy related or unrelated to the first. For that reason, we build long-term follow-up into our studies, to try to identify risk factors for the development of these long-term effects, like second malignancies, cardiac disease, or neurologic toxicity.

Despite these concerns, pharmaceutical companies have been reluctant to test more drugs on children. According to some estimates, only 20 percent of the drugs marketed in the US have been the subject of pediatric clinical trials. Critics of the pharmaceutical industry charge that the reasons are mostly economic: it's expensive to conduct clinical trials, and because relatively few children get cancer or other diseases, the pediatric market is relatively small, and the pharmaceutical companies would be unlikely to recoup their costs. The pharmaceutical industry, on the other hand, maintains that the reasons have more to do with the ethical and legal problems involved in conducting pediatric clinical trials.

In November 1998, the US Food and Drug Administration (FDA) issued new regulations requiring pharmaceutical companies to conduct clinical trials in children "if the product is likely to be used in a substantial number of pediatric patients" or if it's likely to provide a "meaningful therapeutic benefit" compared to existing treatments.[1] These new rules are likely to increase the number of cancer clinical trials for children.

The pharmaceutical companies are correct, however, in asserting that there are important legal and ethical problems in the conduct of clinical trials in children. Because children are considered not to possess a fully mature moral sense, they cannot themselves give informed consent to their participation in clinical trials. After some debate, ethicists have concluded that a child's parents or adult guardians can give informed consent on a child's behalf, provided that (among other requirements) there is a significant possibility that participation in the clinical trial will benefit the individual child. Adults have no such requirement. An adult may choose to participate in a clinical trial even if it is unlikely to benefit him personally.

Dr. Santana notes:

> Depending on where you live in the nation, there are differences in the legal age definition of a "child." In general, the age of consent is eighteen years, but this may vary in different states. If you're not considered an adult, all legal requirements for authority to treat are based on the permission of the parents. In essence, the child doesn't have a major voice in it. Clearly, that presents an ethical issue because as pediatric oncologists, we want our patients to be participants in the process of informed consent. Besides the

age, other factors to consider are emotional maturity, cognitive development, and psychological state. Presenting a clinical trial to a fifteen-year-old is very different than presenting the same trial to a five-year-old.

Although children cannot give informed consent to a clinical trial, both ethical principles and federal law require that the child be asked to "assent" to her participation. The law defines assent as "…a child's affirmative agreement to participate in research. Mere failure to object should not, absent affirmative agreement, be construed as consent."[2] The American Academy of Pediatrics says that assent should be required from any child with an intellectual age of seven or more.[3]

This definition provides little in the way of definitive guidance to parents or to investigators about the operational meaning of assent. William G. Bartholome, MD, MTS, of the University of Kansas Medical Center, believes that assent should involve four elements:[4]

1. The investigator should help the child reach a developmentally appropriate understanding of her condition. He should let her know why she's an appropriate candidate for the clinical trial and why she, rather than some other child, is being asked to participate.

2. Then the investigator should disclose the nature of proposed intervention and what she's likely to experience. He should answer questions such as, "What's going to happen to me?" "What will it feel like?" and "Will I be scared?"

3. The investigator should then assess the child's understanding of the information and the factors influencing her evaluation of the situation.

4. Only after the first three elements of assent are met should the investigator solicit the child's expression of willingness to participate.

This expanded definition of assent does not, however, have the force of law.

Dr. Santana speaks of his experience with children:

From a very legal perspective, the child can never overrule the parents' wishes. As long as the parents are competent people, are acting on behalf of their child, and as long as they've understood the information that's given to them, the parents have the ultimate decision-making vote.

However, we would never administer therapy to a child who physically or emotionally has dissented. We would work with a team of other experts, including social workers, developmental, and behavioral scientists to try to understand why this child is saying no. Many times the reason children say no is a lack of knowledge, or more than anything, that they don't really understand what's going to happen to them, and they're scared. Often, through the process of having other members of the medical team talk to the child and explain what is going to happen, this fear is removed, and dissent is no longer an issue.

If they're saying no because of an extra blood sample or bone-marrow test, or a night in the hospital, those are very concrete things that we can talk about. There may be ways of getting the extra blood samples without having to do a new vein stick every time. There may be a way of getting the extra bone marrow without having additional pain.

If your cancer is advanced

If you have advanced cancer and have been given a poor prognosis with conventional therapy, you have several options regarding clinical trials. But you must make decisions about these options quickly, even if you seem to be doing well at the moment. As Dr. Jablons explains:

People with advanced disease may look good today, but by the time they go around the country, or they do all this research, a month later they might not be feeling as good. Some therapies, which may be relatively stressful or toxic, but which may have the best chance of slowing things or changing things, aren't going to be an option once your performance status drops off.

Among your options are the following:

- You can choose an aggressive and risky early-phase trial aimed at finding a cure.

- You may also be fortunate enough to find a later-phase trial of an especially promising new treatment for your disease.

- As discussed in Chapter 5, *Special Types of Trials*, you may choose supportive-therapy trials designed to better ease your pain or some of the side effects of other therapies.

- You may choose to participate in an early-phase trial, not out of hope of personal benefit, but to help others down the road.

- You may choose not to participate in any clinical trial at all.

Depending on your situation and your personality, any of these options can be valid and rational, and none can be dismissed out of hand.

If you want to take an aggressive course, focus your attention on Phase I and Phase II trials. The NCI's CancerTrials web site (*http://cancertrials.nci.nih.gov/*), which is described more fully in Chapter 4, *How to Find Clinical Trials*, allows you to restrict your search to specific trial phases. As Lydia Cunningham Rising recommended earlier, try to find a trial that's a real departure from the ordinary, one using a promising new drug or an entirely new approach to the disease, rather than an old drug in a new dose or combination.

You may choose to focus not only on how the trial may help you, but also on how your participation might help other people suffering from cancer, whether or not you achieve personal benefit. As discussed previously, Phase I trials are not intended to be therapeutic but instead are intended to determine the drug's safety and its highest tolerated dosage. Only a small percentage of Phase I participants achieve remissions. But all clinical trial participants can take comfort in the fact that they have helped advance medical science. Their generous participation brings us that much closer to an ultimate cure. And when that cure is finally found, as it certainly will be some day, everyone who benefits will owe a debt of gratitude to those who have gone before, those who bravely volunteered.

Not everyone will want to enroll in a trial, and that's all right, too. There comes a time when it might be better to stop looking for innovative medical answers. Dr. Jablons puts it eloquently when he says:

> *For any terminal patient, at the end of it all what matters is the time they have with their loved ones. If they're in pain and there's some experimental trial for pain relief, and you don't have to travel far, and it's not a daily therapy, and it's not in an ICU or a hospital, maybe give it a shot. One thing that is a problem is that patients—and investigators as well—never want to give up.*

No one else can make this personal decision for you. You will most likely want to consult with your family, friends, physicians, and spiritual advisors, but ultimately the decision on whether and when to select or stop treatments must be yours alone.

CHAPTER SEVEN

Evaluating a Clinical Trial

LET'S SAY THAT YOU'VE FOUND one or more candidate clinical trials for your cancer after using the techniques suggested in previous chapters. How do you decide which if any of these trials are for you? If you meet the inclusion criteria and the exclusion criteria don't disqualify you, take a very close look at the informed consent document and—if you can get your hands on it—the trial's protocol. Then you should make sure you get answers to all your questions from the investigators and the clinical trial staff. Finally, you should ask yourself a number of questions before deciding to proceed.

Inclusion and exclusion criteria

The first step is to examine the inclusion criteria, the list of conditions you must meet in order to be considered for participation in a certain clinical trial. It's easy to find the inclusion criteria because it's featured prominently in every clinical trial listing, even if it is very brief.

You'll learn quickly, for example, that a certain clinical trial is looking for people with stage III or stage IV non-small-cell lung cancer. If you have stage II lung cancer, or small-cell lung cancer, or a different kind of cancer entirely, it's pointless even to make a phone call to investigate the trial further, no matter how promising you believe the treatment to be. You simply won't be considered if you don't meet the inclusion criteria.

If you seem to meet the inclusion criteria, the next step is to phone (or to have a friend, relative, or your physician phone) the investigator or the clinical trial coordinator. The first thing she'll do is ask you about your diagnosis. She might have a more detailed list of inclusion criteria than that in the brief clinical trial description. If you still seem eligible, she'll go over the exclusion criteria.

This point is where most potential participants in the clinical trial fall out. In many trials, more than 90 percent of people inquiring about a clinical trial are excluded. Dr. David Jablons, a thoracic surgeon and cancer expert at the University of California, San Francisco, explains:

> The typical clinical trial in cancer is not being done in early stage patients who have the luxury, hopefully, of a long disease-free interval. On the contrary, it's being done on patients with advanced disease who are desperate for any potential, hopeful, experimental therapy. The problem is that the studies usually (but not always) are looking at patients that are freshly diagnosed with advanced disease who haven't seen a lot of therapy to date. It helps keep the data cleaner. If you have a Substance X that you think is really going to be effective, and you start it on patients who have never seen any chemotherapy, who have never had any radiation, then it's pretty easy to say that the result is due to the trial drug. On the other hand, if they've had a bunch of chemotherapy and then you give them Substance X, the data are not as clean.
>
> It's really a paradox. The patients who are the most desperate, the most motivated, and the most interested in innovative therapy plans are usually the patients who have failed conventional therapy.

Some critics of the current system of clinical trials cite overly strict exclusion criteria as the primary cause of the low levels of patient participation.[1] Moreover, they charge that the reasoning behind the desire for strict exclusion criteria might be faulty. The designers of clinical trials want a homogeneous population that has the best possible chance of responding to the experimental treatment. If they succeed in finding that population, clinical trials would take less time and would be less expensive. But that assumes that trial designers can tell in advance which subgroup of patients with a given disease would respond better. There's no evidence that that's the case, and suppose they guess wrong? There's a possibility that they're excluding the very patients who might benefit the most from the new treatment. As Dr. Jablons notes:

Sometimes the rules can be bent. For example, if they've had radiation a year ago, focal radiation might not rule a patient out. But if a person has failed fourteen different drugs as of a month ago, and their disease is rapidly progressing, is that the right person to try a new substance on? It could be, because if you saw a response, you'd say that not only is Substance X effective, but it's effective as a salvage treatment. The problem is that these are rapidly progressing diseases. Clinical disease doesn't always wait for careful, controlled, cautious, trial progression.

Examining the informed consent document

Many people with cancer are so desperate to try anything, or so hopeful that a certain experimental treatment will work, that they're willing to sign the informed consent document without examining it closely. As one patient explains:

I had a specialist in one of the most renowned cancer centers in the world telling me that he recommends this treatment. He's the man. I'm not going to second-guess him.

No matter how hopeful or desperate you are, no matter how anxious you are to start treatment quickly, no matter how much you trust and respect your doctor, it's always a mistake to sign the informed consent before examining it closely, making sure your questions are all answered, and then giving it careful consideration.

Before I started the treatment, informed consent was discussed several different times. The doctor came over when I was still an

inpatient from the surgery and told me he'd like to do CHOP-bleo
[a combination of a standard chemotherapy cocktail called CHOP
with the experimental addition of bleomycin]. He gave me a num-
ber of pamphlets and some typewritten sheets regarding the side
effects of chemotherapy and some literature on CHOP itself and
on what they expected would be the potential side effects of
CHOP-bleo. He asked then if we had any questions. When we got
ready to do it, we went back in one day and did nothing but meet
with the physician assistant, and she went over the informed con-
sent paragraph by paragraph. I kept saying, "Give me the damn
thing. I'll sign it. I want to do this." But she insisted on going over
every bit of it. I certainly understand the reasons for this, but at
that point, I had read it at home. As a cancer patient, I was in the
mindset of, "Do something for me. Let's get rid of this. Let's get on
with it." As it turned out, we signed the papers that day; we went
back the next day and met with the doctor briefly. Two hours later,
I had my first treatment.

Perhaps the best way to understand how to evaluate an informed consent document is to examine an actual one. An informed consent document is reproduced here, interspersed with comments. Certain characteristics of this trial, including the code name of the investigational drug and the identities of the investigator and the sponsoring organizations, have been disguised.

```
A   Randomized,   Double-Blind,   Placebo   Controlled,
Phase  III  Study  of  the  CDK  Inhibitor  ZZ1234  in
Combination  with  Standard  Chemotherapy  in  Patients
Having Advanced Non-Small-Cell Lung Cancer
```

The title alone will give you a great deal of information. You can tell from this title that you won't have a choice about which treatment group you'll be in ("randomized"). You can tell that you won't even be told which treatment group you're in, nor will the investigators know ("double-blind"). You can tell that there's a chance that you'll get an inactive medication instead of the investigational drug ("placebo controlled"). And you can tell that the drug has shown early promise because it has progressed to phase III. Moreover, you can tell what type of drug it is (a "CDK inhibitor"), that the drug will be given together with standard chemotherapy, and that the patients participating in the trial will all have a certain diagnosis ("advanced non-small-cell lung cancer").

It's interesting that the investigational drug is referred to by a number (ZZ1234) instead of a name. That's a clue that the trial might be sponsored by a pharmaceutical company and that the drug is in its early development. Pharmaceutical companies often use numbers for their investigational drugs before the drug is proven in clinical trials. They do this because drug names must be approved by the United States Adopted Names (USAN) Council under the direction of the United States Pharmacopoeia. The USAN considers whether the proposed name is too promotional for the known action of the drug (Cancercurin would probably be unacceptable, for example) and whether the name is too similar to another drug's name, leading to possible confusion in the marketplace. Drug sponsors typically do not go through this step until efficacy and safety have been established in clinical trials.

```
CONSENT TO BE A RESEARCH SUBJECT

PURPOSE AND BACKGROUND

Dr. Jane Smith and associates at the University of
Metropolis Medical Center are evaluating the
effects, safety, and highest dose of a non-approved
investigational drug, ZZ1234. Tablets of ZZ1234 will
be given orally two times a day in combination with
chemotherapy. I will receive one of two doses of
ZZ1234 with chemotherapy, or I will receive placebo
with chemotherapy. I am being asked to take part in
this study because I have lung cancer.
```

This paragraph tells you the name of the principal investigator and her institutional affiliation and gives some more details about the study. It tells you how the drug will be administered ("as an oral tablet taken two times a day") and that you will be given one of two doses of the drug, or a placebo, along with chemotherapy.

Notice however some of the things that are not in the paragraph. (As you will see, they are not to be found in the remainder of the informed consent document either.) You are not told what a CDK inhibitor is, nor why the investigators believe that CDK inhibition might have an effect on cancer. These are areas that you should definitely explore with the investigator before signing the informed consent. If you have researched your cancer and its treatments, you might have an opinion on whether the investigators' theories about CDK inhibition hold water. Even people who don't have the background to conduct this research often find it useful to visualize what the drug is doing to defeat the cancer.

```
Approximately 600 patients will participate in this
study.
```

That's a large number of people. It's unlikely that all these patients can be accommodated at a single institution, so in all likelihood, this is a multicenter trial. It's worthwhile asking about this. (For this particular trial, patients were being recruited at approximately 60 institutions all across the country, and the investigators expected to treat about 10 patients at the University of Metropolis.)

```
PROCEDURES

If I agree to participate in this study, the follow-
ing events will occur:

I will undergo a physical examination, blood and
urine sampling for laboratory evaluations, and an
electrocardiogram (a test to measure my heart
rhythms). My cancer will also be assessed by scans
or other procedures if this has not been done with-
in the past four weeks.

If I am found to be eligible for the study, I will
be determined by chance (like flipping a coin) to
receive either one of the two doses of ZZ1234 with
chemotherapy or chemotherapy with placebo (inactive
```

substance). I will have a 66 percent chance of receiving ZZ1234 and a 33 percent chance of receiving placebo. All patients will receive chemotherapy that is commonly used for cancer like mine. It will not be known by me or my doctor which pill I will receive.

Participants are being randomized so that they receive one of two different doses of ZZ1234 or the placebo, and that makes three arms of the study. If there are equal numbers of patients in each arm, you'd have a 33 percent chance of being in any one arm. That means that you'd have a 66 percent chance of getting one of the doses of the drug and a 33 percent chance of receiving the placebo. Those are pretty good odds.

On the first day of treatment, I will have blood samples (approximately 5 teaspoons) taken for analysis of laboratory values, and I will be asked to answer questions regarding my disease experience. I will begin taking study pills by mouth, every 12 hours (typically at around 9:00 in the morning and 9:00 in the evening) with a glass of water. I will receive my first chemotherapy treatment, which will be a combination of two drugs given by vein over 3 hours. I will continue to take study pills twice daily. I will return about every 3 weeks to have laboratory samples (4 teaspoons) drawn, to receive doses of chemotherapy, and to answer questions about how I feel.

I will also be asked to return to the clinic weekly for 3 weeks during two portions of the study for the purpose of laboratory tests (2 teaspoons each week). My disease will be evaluated monthly by physical exam, blood tests, and chest x-rays; CT scans of the chest will be taken every 6 to 8 weeks as needed. On some of my visits, I will be asked to remain in the clinic for at least 2 hours for collection of blood samples (approximately 4 teaspoons) to measure the amount of drug in my blood.

On one visit, I will be asked to remain in the clinic for at least 6 hours for collection of blood samples (approximately 11 teaspoons), followed the

next day by a visit lasting 4 to 10 hours for collection of blood samples (approximately 3
teaspoons).

This section goes into admirable detail about the exact schedule of
treatment and how often you would be required to come into the
clinic. But it doesn't mention which two drugs constitute the standard chemotherapy treatment. You should definitely find out what
you'll be taking. You might also want to clarify what would happen
if you could not make a clinic visit for some reason. Would that disqualify you from the study entirely, or would they just reschedule
for another day?

Treatment with study pills and chemotherapy will continue until my doctor determines that my disease has
become worse (progressed) or I experience side
effects that require stopping treatment. I will be
asked to return to the clinic periodically until all
side effects are gone.

Depending on my disease evaluation (by physical exam
or radiological assessment), I may be contacted to
answer questions about my disease experience beyond
my time on any of the treatments designated on the
study.

This section discusses when you would stop receiving the investigational drug—if your disease progresses despite treatment or if the
drug appears to be causing unacceptable side effects. But there's no
mention of how long you could continue to receive the drug if your
cancer was responding, and you should certainly clarify that with
the investigator.

If any new information, either good or bad, comes to
the attention of my doctor that may relate to my
willingness to continue to participate, it will be
provided to me. I have been told that if the treatment is no longer in my best interest, the treatment
will be stopped. Should new scientific developments
occur that indicate this treatment is no longer in
my best interest, the treatment will be stopped.

This means that your doctor must tell you if she learns that many patients are experiencing unacceptable side effects from the medication, or that, conversely, the medication seems to be working especially well. It also means that she must inform you of other potential therapies for your cancer that come along, because knowing about them might affect your willingness to continue in this trial. This section seems unclear, however, about what would constitute "new scientific developments...that indicate this treatment is no longer in my best interest," and who would be making that judgment. The document continues:

RISKS AND DISCOMFORTS

Treatment of my cancer is likely to produce side effects and not all effects it will cause are known. My condition will be closely monitored in order to minimize any side effects/risks.

Little is known about ZZ1234. The most common effects that have been seen with ZZ1234 are bitter taste and nausea. It may affect how the body handles other medication, which could have side effects on my liver. It is also possible that we may see other side effects in this study. I will be watched closely to identify and reduce these side effects. As with any experimental drug, there is a small possibility that side effects could be serious or fatal. There have been no major side effect differences between men and women receiving ZZ1234 in previous studies.

The most common side effect of chemotherapy is lowering of the white blood cell count leading to a higher risk of infection. A low platelet count can develop leading to a higher risk of bleeding. A low red blood cell count leading to anemia will occur. Hair loss and muscle or joint pains are often seen. Less common effects include nerve damage leading to numbness or tingling, hearing loss, muscle weakness, seizures, and possible mouth sores and inflammation of the colon. Allergic reactions can occur. These can be severe. Nausea, vomiting, palpitations, and changes in blood pressure have also been seen.

> My treatments may be delayed and doses of these drugs
> reduced if the side effects are severe. If my blood
> counts fall very low, I may need to come into the
> hospital and transfusions may be required.
>
> Muscle pains after chemotherapy usually last for a
> few days. Hair loss will usually come back after
> treatment is stopped. Other medicines may be given
> to keep side effects under control.

Always examine the lists of side effects very carefully. One striking thing in this document is how mild the stated side effects of ZZ1234 are compared to the standard—and widely used—chemotherapy regimen.

> This study may be hazardous to an unborn or nursing
> child. There is insufficient medical information to
> determine whether there are significant risks to a
> nursing infant or to a fetus carried by a mother who
> is participating in this study. Effective birth con-
> trol measures must be used by all participants or
> their sexual partners while participating in this
> study. Nursing mothers must discontinue nursing. If
> I become pregnant, I will be disqualified from the
> study. If I think I might be pregnant at any time
> during the study, I should tell my doctor.

Not only does the investigational drug present unknown hazards, but many standard chemotherapeutic agents are known to be harmful to unborn or nursing children. For this reason, women of childbearing age must be especially careful to prevent pregnancy, and nursing mothers must discontinue nursing.

> The risks of drawing blood include temporary discom-
> fort from the needle stick, bruising, and rarely,
> infection.

Here's an example of the informed consent document being overly conscientious in listing every possible side effect. It's practically unheard of for medical technologists to give you informed consent about the side effects of needle sticks before drawing blood! It's better, however, that the informed consent err on the side of providing too many warnings than too few.

```
I will be assigned to a treatment program by chance.
The treatment I receive may prove to be less effec-
tive or to have more side effects than the other
study treatments or than other available treatments.
This will not be known until after the study is com-
pleted and the data have been analyzed.
```

This is a risk in all clinical trials. All participants in clinical trials take the chance that the study medication may be worse than the standard treatment. There's no way to know this ahead of time; if there were, there'd be no point in conducting the study.

FINANCIAL RISKS

```
The costs of all visits, treatments, and tests
described in the Procedures section of this consent
form will be billed to me or my insurance, with the
exception of study pills and procedures or special
tests that are required as a part of this study but
are not a part of my standard medical care. These
tests will be provided to me at no cost through an
agreement between the sponsor, Acme Pharmaceuticals,
Inc., and my doctor. I, or my insurance company, will
be responsible for the cost of medications or proce-
dures associated with the routine medical care of my
cancer, including any complications of my underlying
illness. Insurance companies and other third-party
payers for health care have sometimes refused to pay
the costs of treatment for patients in research stud-
ies, in which case I am responsible for all costs.
```

This paragraph reveals the name of the drug company sponsoring the study and points out that the company will pay for the study medication, as well as associated procedures and tests. However, it will not pay for the standard care of your cancer. Before entering a study, you should determine whether your insurance company or health maintenance organization will pick up these other costs. For more information on this aspect of clinical trials, see Chapter 9, *Financial Issues*.

Along with the risks of participating, informed consent documents
also list the benefits. It's characteristic that the list of benefits is
shorter and much less specific than the list of risks.

Typically, this section will also include information on other available clinical trials for your cancer at the host institution. Pay careful
attention to the section on alternatives, which emphasizes that you
genuinely do have a choice about whether to participate in a given
clinical trial.

Few cancer clinical trials provide payment or reimbursement to
participants. Occasionally, transportation costs or car fare might be
covered, and sometimes additional payments are even made. But
these tend to be reserved for healthy volunteers participating in
phase I studies.

This section discusses what will happen if you suffer serious side effects of the study. You will want to ask the investigator what is meant by "...may be covered...depending on a number of factors." What are those factors? How will it be determined whether you were injured by the study medication or by the standard chemotherapy? Who makes that determination? Note that only treatment, and not "any other form of compensation for injury," is provided. This means that you won't be compensated for pain and suffering, for example, and you will not be entitled to any kind of cash award if something untoward happens.

QUESTIONS

Don't sign the informed consent until all your questions have been answered. If other questions arise later, don't be shy about contacting Dr. Smith.

CONFIDENTIALITY

representatives from the Food and Drug Administration (FDA) and Acme Pharmaceuticals, Inc. (the sponsor), may be allowed to see my records to check on the study.

Although you do lose some privacy by participating in a clinical trial, you needn't worry about your name appearing in an article in (for example) the *Journal of the American Medical Association*. You might want to ask the investigator whether she plans to mention individual patients in the scientific article describing this study, and if so, how she will conceal your identity.

CONSENT

Participation in research is voluntary. I have the right to withdraw from the study at any time, and withdrawing will not jeopardize my future medical care. My participation may be ended at any time with or without my consent. My doctor may discontinue my participation in this study if I experience excessive side effects or deterioration in my health or I do not follow the study procedures. The sponsor of the study, Acme Pharmaceuticals, Inc., may also terminate my participation in this study if new findings indicate that continuation of my participation would be potentially dangerous to my health. The sponsor may terminate the study for other reasons unrelated to the purpose of this research study. If I wish to participate, I should sign below. I have been given a signed copy of this document and a copy of the Experimental Subject's Bill of Rights to keep.

Both you and the investigator may terminate your participation in the trial at any time. You might want to consider what might make you leave the trial prematurely. And you should ask the investigator what would cause her to drop you from the study. How much of a deterioration in your health would be enough, for example? How closely must you follow study procedures? Would you be dropped for forgetting to take a single dose or for taking the dose an hour late?

EXPERIMENTAL SUBJECT'S BILL OF RIGHTS

The rights below are the rights of every person who is asked to be in a research study. As an experimental subject, I have the following rights:

1. To be told what the study is trying to find out,

2. To be told what will happen to me and whether any of the procedures, drugs, or devices is different from what would be used in standard practice,

3. To be told about the frequent and/or important risks, side effects, or discomforts of the things that will happen to me for research purposes,

4. To be told if I can expect any benefit from participating, and, if so, what the benefit might be,

5. To be told of the other choices I have and how they may be better or worse than being in the study,

6. To be allowed to ask any questions concerning the study both before agreeing to be involved and during the course of the study,

7. To be told what sort of medical treatment is available if any complications arise,

8. To refuse to participate at all or to change my mind about participation after the study has started. This decision will not affect my right to receive the care I would receive if I were not in the study,

9. To receive a copy of the signed and dated consent form,

10. To be free of pressure when considering whether I wish to agree to be in the study.

If I have other questions, I should ask the researcher or the research assistant. In addition, I may contact the Institutional Review Board, which is concerned with the protection of volunteers in research projects. I may reach the committee office by calling 555-5555 from 8:00 a.m. to 5:00 p.m., Monday to Friday, or by writing to the Institutional Review Board, University of Metropolis, Metropolis, CA 90000.

Not every informed consent document will have a separately enumerated "Experimental Subject's Bill of Rights," which is a legislative requirement that has been enacted only in certain states. This is California's version. In other states, some or all of the rights listed here will be incorporated into the main body of the consent document. If you believe that any of your rights have been violated, you should contact the investigator or the Institutional Review Board immediately.

Examining the protocol document

Because the informed consent document often lacks crucial information, the savvy patient will obtain a copy of the trial's protocol. The protocol is a lengthy and highly technical document that contains every scientific detail of the clinical trial.

The protocol contains sections explaining the full scientific rationale of the study. Why do the investigators expect this compound to be active in cancer? What is its chemical makeup? What does it do in the test tube? How did it perform in animal studies? How did it perform in earlier phases of human testing?

The protocol also contains sections explaining the detailed conduct of the present study. How many patients and what kind of patients will be enrolled? What are the detailed inclusion and exclusion criteria? What drugs will be administered, and when? What tests will be administered, and when? How is the clinical staff supposed to respond to certain side effects and other contingencies? What would cause them to drop you from the study?

All of these questions—and many more—will be answered in the protocol for those patients willing to slog through language intended not for patients but for scientists and regulatory agencies.

Joyce R. Niblack speaks from experience:

> Before anybody goes into a clinical trial, they should get and read a copy of the protocol. If there's something they don't understand, they need to ask questions. And if there's anything in there that's not acceptable to them, they need to negotiate. For example, in the first clinical trial I participated in, the protocol required a bone marrow biopsy once a month. Now, these are not fun. My doctor asked me, "Do you want these once a month?" and I said, "Hell no!" He said, "Well, I think it's insane." So I refused to agree to that. I negotiated through my doctor. He felt it was absolute nonsense to require it once a month. Interferon works slowly on the marrow, so he didn't think in any event you would see a big change from month to month. He told them he would be happy to monitor me through blood work, and he would give them bone marrow slides every three months, and that was it. My disease is so rare that I don't think there were many people falling off the tree saying, "Let me in your study," so they agreed.

Steve Dunn offers another reason to examine the protocol:

> I think the most valuable thing in the protocol is to read about the prior history of this thing, and why they think it's promising, because that will tell you what the worth of the trial is. What most people hear about is the rate: "This has a 30 percent response rate in previous trials." But what you really are looking for in a Phase I or Phase II trial is that it makes the cancer go away and makes the cancer stay away. The problem is that there are an awful lot of treatments where the cancer might go away, but it'll grow back. What's really promising is if it looks like the responses are long-lasting and some of these people are getting quality time.

Steve points out that there's no way of telling what kind of valuable nuggets of information you might find in a careful perusal of the protocol. He believes that one of the things he learned might have helped him derive the maximum benefit from his trial.

When I read the protocol document for my trial, I found that they were very interested in neurological side effects and that they would withhold doses of the treatment if you had any. Knowing this helped me when I was in the treatment because they would offer me pain pills, and they would offer me compazine [a major tranquilizer that also decreases nausea], and they would offer me sleeping pills. Guess what? All of these things sedate you, and if you get into enough of a stupor with all of it, they would withhold doses. So I went really light on all of that stuff. You can't predict what little facts you might learn in the protocol that would help you get through the treatment better.

The major problem with the protocol is that it's written not at the eighth-grade level or below, as are most informed consent documents. On the contrary, it's written for people with MDs or PhDs. To make some sense out of all of the technical jargon, use the resources suggested in Chapter 4, *How to Find Clinical Trials*.

In *Childhood Leukemia: A Guide for Families, Friends, & Caregivers*, Nancy Keene lists some of the reasons that parents will want to obtain protocol documents related to their children. These reasons apply equally well to adults enrolled in cancer clinical trials.

Admittedly, for some parents, the full protocol could be overwhelming or boring. There are many parents, however, who throw themselves into research to better understand their child's illness. These parents may benefit from having a copy of the study document for several reasons. First, it provides a description of all the clinical trials that preceded the present one and explains the reasons the investigators designed this particular study. Secondly, it provides detailed descriptions of drug reactions, which comforts many parents who worry that their child is the only one exhibiting extreme responses to some drugs. Thirdly, motivated parents who have only one protocol to keep track of occasionally prevent serious errors in treatment. Physicians treat scores of children on dozens of protocols and sometimes make mistakes. And finally, for parents who are adrift in the world of cancer treatment, it can return a bit of control over their child's life. It gives the parents a job to do: monitor their child's treatment.

Despite the value of the protocol document to the patient, it's not always easy to pry it loose from the investigators or their staffs. There are several reasons that they may be reluctant to show you the protocol. Sometimes it's misplaced paternalism. You have no medical training, they'll say, and the protocol is far too complicated for you to understand. You can counter that objection by pointing out that you or a trusted family member has been forced into becoming an expert in one narrow area of medicine, that you realize you might not understand every word, but that you'll ask questions if something concerns or confuses you.

Another reason the staff might be reluctant to give you the protocol is that it's a pain in the neck for them. Most protocols are 70 to 100 pages long, and some are even longer than that. They tend to reside in thick, loose-leaf notebooks, and it's not an insignificant task to photocopy something like that. They might say, hey, we're running 50 patients through this trial, and the protocol is 100 pages. Suppose everybody asks for a copy? You can answer this objection by pointing out that you're not 50 people, you're only one person who needs one copy. And you or a relative can offer to work the photocopier or take it to a copy shop if staff members don't have the time. You can also offer to read their copy in their offices, but if you choose that option, be sure not to let yourself be rushed. Take your time, and come with a pencil and paper so you can take notes.

A more serious obstacle to obtaining the protocol can present itself in some trials sponsored by pharmaceutical companies. Because these companies are often concerned about details of their new wonder drug leaking to their competitors, they often insist that investigators sign confidentiality agreements. This prohibits investigators from showing the protocol or even discussing certain details of the trial with others. If a member of the clinical research staff tells you that you can't have the protocol for this reason, you should immediately ask to speak to the principal investigator because people lower on the totem pole usually don't have the authority to make exceptions to the confidentiality rule.

Explain to the investigator that there simply isn't enough information in the informed consent document for you to make a fully informed decision about participating in the trial. He will likely counter with an offer to answer any questions you have. Tell him that although you appreciate his willingness to answer your questions, until you've had a chance to read the protocol, you won't even be able to formulate proper questions. The investigator may well conclude that he has an ethical obligation to release the protocol to you despite the confidentiality agreement. If he's still hesitant, offer to sign a confidentiality agreement yourself. Dr. David Jablons offers his view: "I think that patients should have complete *carte blanche* access to the protocol, within the bounds set by the company."

If the investigator still won't budge, ask to see just part of the protocol. The introductory sections tend to be the parts that are most valuable to clinical trial participants, and the investigator might be more willing to show you this one section than the whole thing. If even that suggestion won't move him, contact someone on the Institutional Review Board (IRB), whose telephone number will appear on the informed consent document. Explain to the IRB member why you want to see the protocol. The IRB might direct the investigator to make an exception to the confidentiality rule.

Throughout this process, be pleasant and polite but firm in your resolve to obtain the protocol. It would most likely be counterproductive to become angry or confrontational, and it would be an especially bad idea to suggest that the investigator was withholding the protocol because he had something to hide.

If you are unable to obtain the protocol even after applying your best efforts, you might want to draw up an especially long and detailed list of questions for the investigator. Be sure to ask for all the information you expect you might have learned by reading the protocol.

Getting questions answered

No matter how desperate you are to enter a clinical trial, you should make sure all your questions are answered before proceeding. Lydia Cunningham Rising tells a story that illustrates this point nicely. When Rising was searching for a clinical trial for her ex-husband, she found only two physicians doing research on his type of brain cancer. One of them was very hard to reach, and when she finally did get him on the phone:

> He was very evasive. He would not answer my questions. When I tried to find out how many people he'd treated and how they did, he would never give me a straight answer. The other doctor told me that he'd treated nine patients and two were still alive after a few years. Joe would be number ten. He just laid it all out, so we went there. Six or seven years later, I came across a journal article written by the doctor who had been evasive. Of the sixty-five patients he treated, not one survived longer than a year. Now you know why the man didn't tell me. If anyone is being evasive, he may well have something to hide.

It's a good idea to bring a tape recorder to meetings with the investigator or trial administrators in which you ask these questions. It can be difficult to take notes while listening with full concentration, and a tape will contain a full record of everything that was said. Be sure to inform everyone in the room that you intend to tape the conversation; in many states, it's illegal to record people without their knowledge. If you don't have access to a tape recorder, go with a friend or family member and ask that person to take notes so you can devote your full attention to the discussion.

Questions to ask your doctor and the trial's principal investigator

- What is the purpose of the study?

- What is the theory behind this new treatment?

- How many people have received this experimental treatment?

- How did their cancers respond? Did they have complete or partial remissions? How long did these remissions last?

- What would my prognosis be without any treatment at all?

- What would my prognosis be with the standard treatment?

- What kind of side effects have you noticed with the experimental treatment? How severe were those side effects? How many patients experienced them?

- Can you put me in touch with other patients participating in this study?

- If I experience side effects, will you give me medication to alleviate them?

- How many patients have dropped out of the study?

- Why did they drop out?

- What would cause you to drop me from this study?

- Suppose I decide to pursue alternative treatments, such as herbal remedies or massage, in addition to the experimental treatment. Will that disqualify me?

- Suppose I seem to be responding to the treatment when the study ends. Will I be able to continue receiving the treatment?

- What are my chances of receiving a placebo?

- Will I be randomized into one of the treatment arms? Please describe in detail all of the arms of the study.

- Who is reviewing this trial? How often is it being reviewed? Who will be monitoring patient safety?

- How will I know if the treatment is working?

- Suppose patients in one of the arms seem to be doing significantly better than the others. Will we all get a chance to switch into that arm?

- Will I know which arm I'm in, or will the trial be blinded?

- Is this a multicenter trial? If so, where else is it being conducted? What is the total number of patients in this trial, and how many of them are being seen at this institution? Are any of the other institutions closer to my home or easier to get to, and if so, can I be seen there?

- What other clinical trials on my kind of cancer are being conducted at this institution or elsewhere? Are any of them especially promising? Do you think this one is better than those? If so, why?

- How long will the study last? Is this longer or shorter than the standard treatment?

- Who will be in charge of my care? Will I be able to see my own doctor?

- Will I receive long-term follow-up care?

- What happens if I suffer serious harm as a result of this trial? Who would pay for the care I might need?

- If a member of your family had the same kind of cancer I do, would you recommend this trial?

- In your opinion, am I better off enrolling in this trial now or waiting a while for something more promising to come along?

Questions to ask those administering the trial

- When will the trial start?

- How often will I have to come to the clinic?

- Can a local laboratory or my personal physician perform any of these tests so I don't have to come all the way down here every time?

- What medical records do you need my personal physician or my HMO to provide?

- Have insurance companies and HMOs been willing to pay for treatment under this study? Will you help me deal with my insurance company? Will you clearly explain to them which parts of this study involve standard treatment—which they should pay for—and which parts are experimental?

- Will I have to pay anything for the experimental parts of the clinical trial?

- Who is sponsoring the clinical trial?

- Whom can I contact if I have any difficulty with this trial? What are their phone numbers, fax numbers, email addresses, and mailing addresses?

Questions to ask yourself

- Given my prognosis, how much of a risk am I willing to take on an experimental treatment?

- Am I sure I fully understand all of my alternatives? What would happen if I did nothing? What would happen if I went with the standard treatment? What would happen if I decided to go with alternative therapies?

- What is the best-case scenario if I participate in this trial? What is the worst-case scenario?

- What would I consider a successful outcome?

- Is the treatment likely to improve my quality of life, the length of my life, or both?

- What level of side effects would cause me to drop out of the trial?

- Is there anything else that might cause me to leave the trial prematurely?

- Suppose I were randomized to the standard-treatment arm of the study. Would that cause me to drop out and search for another trial?

- Have I had all my questions answered? If not, was anybody being evasive? Do I trust the investigator?

- Do I trust the trial's sponsor?

- Do I trust my insurance company/HMO to pay its fair share of the trial's costs?

- How difficult will it be for me to get to the hospital or clinic for my treatment?

- Am I better off enrolling in this trial now or waiting a while for something more promising to come along?

CHAPTER EIGHT

Administration of Clinical Trials

"YOU CAN'T TELL THE PLAYERS without a scorecard," shouts the ball-park vendor. If you're considering a clinical trial, it's important to understand who the players are and what positions they play in the complex—and deadly serious—game of cancer research.

Food and Drug Administration

The overall responsibility for the evaluation and approval of new cancer treatments and the conduct of cancer clinical trials lies with the US Food and Drug Administration (FDA) and in most cases with the FDA's Center for Drug Evaluation and Research (CDER). (Medical devices are the province of the FDA's Center for Devices and Radiological Health.) There is a great deal of detailed information about the FDA's activities on its helpful web site, *http://www.fda.gov/*.

The path to approval for a new cancer therapy is a complex one. What follows is a highly abbreviated summary. For more particulars, see CDER's web site at *http://www.fda.gov/cder/* and especially the "CDER Handbook" at *http://www.fda.gov/cder/handbook/*.

Before clinical trials can even begin, the sponsor—an individual, partnership, corporation, government agency, manufacturer, or scientific institution—must submit an Investigational New Drug (IND) application to CDER. CDER reviews the preclinical data about the drug's safety and effectiveness, it reviews information related to how the drug is manufactured, it reviews the proposed protocols for the clinical trial, and it reviews the qualifications of the clinical investigators. If CDER judges all these factors to be acceptable, it will permit clinical trials to proceed. Technically, however, what CDER grants when it approves an IND is an exemption to the federal statute that prohibits unapproved drugs from being shipped across state lines.

With the IND in hand, the sponsor conducts clinical trials. Once Phase III clinical trials are completed successfully, the sponsor submits a New Drug Application (NDA) to CDER. NDAs are massive filings, occupying many thousands of pages containing every detail about the scientific and clinical aspects of the new treatment and the clinical trials that establish its safety and effectiveness. Records of each individual participant in all the clinical trials are included. CDER reviews every aspect of the NDA, and the application is also reviewed by an FDA advisory committee—a group of outside experts. If the NDA passes all those hurdles, and the advisory committee recommends approval, the FDA grants the manufacturer the right to market the drug for certain conditions.

In 1996, the FDA undertook several initiatives designed to improve patient access to new cancer therapies. The most important of these initiatives allowed sponsors to demonstrate a new treatment's effectiveness using a "surrogate marker." Previously, sponsors had to demonstrate actual increases in survival time for a new therapy to be approved. Because it takes quite a long time to accumulate survival-time statistics, the approval process often moved slowly. Beginning in 1996, the FDA began approving treatments when the sponsor merely demonstrated tumor shrinkage as an early indicator of the treatment's effectiveness, thus speeding the approval process.

The management of clinical trials

The conduct of clinical trials differ somewhat depending on who initiates, who manages, and who funds them. Cancer clinical trials are typically initiated and managed either by scientists at academic institutions, by pharmaceutical companies, or by the National Cancer Institute (NCI). They are usually funded either by pharmaceutical companies or the NCI. (Some cancer clinical trials are also funded by the Department of Veterans Affairs or by the Department of Defense.)

One common scenario occurs when a clinical trial is initiated by an individual investigator or small group of investigators at an academic medical center. It obtains funding in the form of grants from the NCI or from pharmaceutical companies. Often investigators band together into what are known as "cooperative groups," which manage multicenter trials.

These cooperative groups differ in structure and research focus. Some, such as the Southwest Oncology Group, bring together investigators in a certain geographical region. Others, such as the Radiation Therapy Oncology Group, study a specific type of cancer therapy. Others, such as the Pediatric Oncology group, concentrate on a certain type of patient. Still others, such as the Gynecologic Oncology Group, focus on a group of related cancers.

Dr. Richard A. Gams, chief scientific officer of Prologue Research International, Inc., is an oncologist who has been associated with several academic institutions and several pharmaceutical companies. He explains how management differs when a trial is being done for FDA submission:

> In a clinical trial done in an academic medical center, generally the NCI or a company may simply turn over a therapeutic substance to academic investigators, who will be fully responsible for the design and conduct of the trial. They will do their own data management; they will do their own reporting. This will result in a publication in a scientific journal. In a trial designed for FDA submission, however, the sponsor will usually write the protocol, recruit an investigator to participate in the protocol, file the protocol with the FDA, actually send its own personnel out to the site to

monitor the conduct of the trial, bring the data back to the company, do all the final analyses, help the investigator to publish the study, and submit the final study reports to the FDA.

It used to be that academic scientists initiated nearly all clinical trials, even the ones that were funded by pharmaceutical companies. But in the 1980s, the FDA began to take a much closer look at the data submitted as part of new drug applications. Dr. Gams explains:

> I think in the 1980s we moved from what I would call the "grant era" of doing clinical trials—where someone would give an investigator money to do what the investigator wanted to do—to the "contract era"—where we would give investigators money to do what we wanted them to do. The FDA began taking a much more critical look at the data. Pharmaceutical companies began recognizing that university investigators often were not as meticulous in meeting all the requirements of the regulatory environment. Pharmaceutical companies ultimately recognized that rather than depend on the investigators to initiate the studies, and rather than depending on the cooperative groups to identify the investigators, they began to control the trial completely from within the company. They had to develop a medical department that consisted of physicians, clinical research associates who would actually go out and visit the sites and monitor the studies, information systems departments, biostatisticians, etc.

Dr. David Jablons notes:

> Whether a trial is sponsored by a drug company or by the NCI, in reality the conduct of the trial is no different. It has to be the same rigorously controlled environment; otherwise you can never interpret the data at the end of the day. The only things that are a little different are the motivations to a certain extent, what kind of questions different groups are answering. Drug companies usually have very focused questions regarding certain stages of patients and what the efficacy end points are. NCI or other government-

sponsored trials are sometimes a little more open ended. Drug companies need to have very focused questions because clinical trials are enormously expensive. They have to choose carefully and wisely where their likely efficacy will be seen in the quickest period of time.

Large pharmaceutical companies were hard hit during the economic recession of the early 1990s. They began downsizing, and one of the areas where they economized was in their newly created medical departments. But they found that they still needed to have a great deal of control over certain aspects of clinical trials. To provide this service, freestanding companies, called "contract research organizations" (CROs), started springing up.

At first the CROs were highly specialized. One would provide biostatistical advice, helping the pharmaceutical companies analyze the data from clinical trials. Another would provide people called clinical research associates who would go to the academic institution and monitor the conduct of the trial. Still another would specialize in regulatory affairs, helping the company compile its submissions to the FDA.

Eventually, full-service CROs began to emerge. When a pharmaceutical company had a drug that was ready for clinical trials, it would hire a single CRO to manage the trials from start to finish. The CRO would write the protocol, it would recruit researchers at a number of hospitals, it would help recruit patients, it would oversee the conduct of the trial, it would collect and analyze the data, and it would prepare the FDA submission.

Many cancer clinical trials are conducted this way today. Interestingly, few patients realize this because the CRO is often invisible. Typically, your direct contact will be with the individual investigator, and if you ask, you'll be told which pharmaceutical company is sponsoring the trial. Unless you ask, however, you probably would never realize that there was an entirely separate entity running all the day-to-day details of the trial. This is not necessarily a bad thing. For the everyday details of a clinical trial, you'll be dealing directly with the investigator and his staff. In the event of serious problems that can't be handled at that level, you'll be dealing with the Institutional Review Board (IRB). For problems that can't be resolved at the IRB level, you can contact the FDA. There are circumstances in which you might want to deal with the pharmaceutical company sponsoring the trial. Although it might be nice to know about any CROs that are involved in the trial, from a patient's point of view, it is rarely necessary.

As mentioned earlier, pharmaceutical companies don't sponsor all trials. Other clinical trials are sponsored by the NCI and conducted by NCI-funded "extramural" (outside) institutions—often major medical centers. But not all trials are conducted by physicians at large hospitals. In 1983, the NCI established the Community Clinical Oncology Program (CCOP), a way for physicians who are not located at academic medical centers to participate in clinical trials. Physicians participating in the CCOP will establish an affiliation with either a cooperative group or a major cancer center, and they enroll their patients in clinical trials whose protocols were developed by their affiliates. The advantage of the CCOP is that it brings the possibility of participating in clinical trials to patients who might be a long way from a major cancer center. If you're not being treated at a major cancer center, you should ask your oncologist whether he's part of the CCOP.

Still other NCI clinical trials are "intramural"—conducted at the NCI Clinical Center in Bethesda, Maryland. According to Dale Shoemaker, chief of the regulatory affairs branch of NCI's Cancer Therapy Evaluation Program, the NCI often conducts research on agents that might not currently have a pharmaceutical collaborator. If clinical trials reveal this agent to be promising in cancer treatment, the NCI will advertise for a pharmaceutical company able to shepherd the drug through the FDA's approval process and able also to market the drug once it's approved.

Investigators and their staff

Every clinical trial at every institution has one individual who is primarily responsible for the conduct of that trial. This person is called the principal investigator (PI), and he is almost always a medical doctor. Depending on the treatment being tested, the principal investigator may be an oncologist, surgeon, radiologist, or anesthesiologist. In a multicenter trial, there will be a PI at each participating institution.

The PI may or may not be the individual directly providing your medical care. Sometimes two or more physicians at an institution have equal responsibility for the conduct of a trial. When that's the case, they're referred to as co-PIs. Other times the person providing your medical care will be a subordinate of the PI.

You'll also be dealing with several people who are not physicians. Many PIs employ a physician assistant or a nurse (sometimes called a research nurse or a nurse coordinator) to handle most of the administrative details involved in clinical trials. Gregory T. David works for Dr. David Jablons at the University of California, San Fransisco (UCSF) in this capacity. As thoracic surgery nurse coordinator, Gregory's would be the first voice you heard if you phoned regarding one of the trials Dr. Jablons is running. During that call Gregory would ask you questions to determine whether you were eligible for the trial, and he'd arrange your initial and subsequent visits. He'd also work with you and your insurance company to obtain reimbursement, and he'd handle a thousand other administrative details.

Another person you're likely to encounter is a clinical research associate (CRA). Employed sometimes by the PI and sometimes by the pharmaceutical company or contract research organization, the CRA must manage the mountain of paperwork generated in each clinical trial and ensure that every aspect of the protocol is followed to the letter and clearly documented.

Institutional Review Boards

Federal law requires that every institution that conducts research on human beings and also receives federal funds must maintain an Institutional Review Board (IRB)—a committee charged with overseeing that research.[1] Although most of these committees are indeed called IRBs, some have different names. For example, UCSF calls its IRB the Committee for Human Research.

The law is very specific about the makeup of the IRB. The IRB must have at least five members of varying backgrounds who are knowledgeable about human research. This committee must not be composed of all men or all women and must be sufficiently diverse—by race, gender, cultural background, and sensitivity to community attitudes—to "promote respect for its advice and counsel in safeguarding the rights and welfare of human subjects." Every IRB must include at least one member who is not affiliated with the institution in any way. This person is generally referred to as the public member. And every IRB must include both scientists and non-scientists.

Although only five members are required, most major research institutions have far more IRB members than that. In part this reflects a desire to obtain a wide range of views, but it's also an effort to divide the large workload among a greater number of people. For example, UCSF's IRB typically has between thirteen and eighteen members, according to Sharon K. Friend, the university's IRB administrator. The UCSF Committee for Human Research is usually made up of the following:

- One to three oncologists

- An AIDS specialist

- A pediatrician

- A radiologist or nuclear-medicine specialist

- A pharmacist who specializes in investigational new drugs

- A clinical nurse specialist
- A behavioral scientist
- A psychiatrist
- An anesthesiologist
- An internist
- A surgeon or obstetrician/gynecologist
- An epidemiologist or biostatistician
- The public member

At UCSF, these committee members are appointed for two-year terms. They meet once a week for about two hours, and except for the committee chairs, they are not paid for their service. Seven to eight full-time staff members serve the committee's administrative needs.

Federal law is also very specific about the IRB's job. It gives the IRB authority to approve, require modification to, or disapprove all research involving human subjects. Moreover, the IRB is charged with overseeing informed consent and with conducting annual reviews of all ongoing human research.

In practice, every investigator who wants to conduct a clinical trial must submit the detailed protocol, as well as the proposed informed consent documents, to the IRB for approval. The IRB will conduct a close examination of both the scientific validity and the patient-protection aspects of the trial. Some institutions have a separate committee, often called the Protocol Review Committee, that concentrates on the scientific aspects of the protocol.

Dr. Victor Santana notes:

> In the past year, we have rejected one protocol out of 25 new ones submitted for review. That specific proposal was something very risky, and there was no direct benefit to the patient. I would

say that 85 percent of protocols require some modification, either in the protocol document itself or in the informed consent, upon IRB review.

Sharon K. Friend discusses some of the process of review:

There's a lot of attention paid to the who, when, where, why, and how of the consent. We wouldn't want to see somebody in labor asked to give consent. There's a lot of discussion about when, in terms of surgery, a patient would get talked to about a project. Is it okay the morning of surgery? Who is the best person to be talking to the patient? What if they're trying to recruit people through medical records? Will they be sending out letters or making phone calls or putting up notices? We'd want to see all that. If there's a national ad campaign, we'd like to see the video or the text. The main thing we look at with ads and recruitment materials is that they're not over-promising benefits.

IRBs encourage patients and their families to come to them with any questions, concerns, or difficulties with clinical trials that the investigator or her staff have been unable to address to the patient's satisfaction. Dr. Santana, who is not only a pediatric oncologist but who is also the chairman of the IRB at St. Jude's, makes sure that every informed consent contains a telephone number that parents and patients can call with questions. At UCSF, the informed consent contains the IRB's phone number and address. About the IRB, Sharon Friend says:

We are the one place that's 100 percent for the subjects. If somebody calls us with a problem, then we're on the phone right away with the investigator, and they take our calls very seriously.

On the other hand, the IRB's attention to detail can prove frustrating to patients and investigators alike. Depending on the institution, it can take several weeks for the IRB to approve a protocol, even one that requires no changes. If the IRB asks the investigator to make a series of changes to the protocol or to the informed consent, it can be months before the clinical trial can begin. One investigator expressed his frustration this way:

> *Our IRB is relatively slow and relatively difficult. It can take three months. It can take six months. It can take a year. Usually the stumbling blocks are not major philosophical things. They're detail-oriented, and they may be driven by semantics or personal agendas. I can't tell you the amount of* Sturm und Drang *that's generated over the wording of consents. It's a bunch of crap. I think there should be one standardized, nationwide consent, to which you'd add the individual experimental details. It's a huge problem. These patients aren't waiting around. They're dying quickly. It's very frustrating from the perspective of trying to be an effective machine for clinical trials, to attract the best, the hottest, the most interesting science, and to bring it to the clinical arena.*

Not every IRB is part of an academic institution. With the advent of contract research organizations has come the freestanding IRB— for-profit companies that will review protocols for a price. When a CRO manages a clinical trial, it will often recruit a disparate group of oncologists in private practice to enroll patients and to administer the experimental treatment. Because none of these physicians will be part of an institution that maintains an IRB, the CRO will hire a freestanding IRB to review the protocol.

One might worry that a freestanding IRB would be likely to rubberstamp any protocol handed to it by the company that's also paying its bills. But Dr. Richard A. Gams, chief scientific officer of Prologue Research International, Inc., an Ohio-based CRO that specializes in cancer trials, denies that that's a problem. He notes that freestanding IRBs are subject to the same federal laws as are institutional IRBs, and that in any case institutional IRBs have similar potential conflicts of interest. After all, most members of an institutional IRB are employed by the institution, and they have an interest in approving protocols so that the institution can garner the funding and the prestige that come with conducting clinical research. Despite that, notes Dr. Gams, institutional IRBs are anything but push-overs, and he maintains that this is true of freestanding IRBs as well.

Multicenter trials

It used to be that a single investigator would initiate a clinical trial and conduct it solely at his own institution. These days, however, few clinical trials are under the control of individual investigators, and more clinical trials are being conducted at several institutions simultaneously.

These are known as multicenter trials, and they have several advantages over single-center trials. As the saying goes, many hands make light work, and multicenter trials decrease the burden on any single institution. Instead of having to find and treat hundreds of patients, a single institution may only have to deal with a few dozen. With several institutions in different regions of the country all searching for participants, patients can be enrolled in the trial more quickly, and the trial can be concluded and its results determined more promptly. Because patients will be recruited from widely separated geographical areas, the treatment will be given to a group of people that is not overly homogeneous and is more representative of the population at large. From the patients' perspective, multicenter trials increase the likelihood that an innovative treatment might be available locally, so travel may present less of a problem.

Multicenter trials present their own set of problems. When you have a number of different physicians with different levels of expertise and different styles, all treating participants in the same clinical trial, there's a danger that the data at different sites may not be comparable. Dr. Jablons explains:

> The problem in multiple sites is you have to make sure there's good quality control. It's not that the doctors aren't good at all

these academic institutions, but for example, if you're not trained to stage patients the appropriate way, earlier stage patients are thrown into the mix, and that skews the data.

Another danger of multicenter trials is that no single institution, and thus no single IRB, has control over the trial.[2] Suppose a trial is being conducted at a dozen institutions. Typically, a single protocol will be circulated to each of the institutions. The principal investigator at each institution will submit that protocol to his IRB. If eleven IRBs at eleven institutions approve the protocol, there is enormous pressure on that last IRB to approve the protocol as well, even if there are serious ethical or scientific concerns. Some IRBs find themselves in uncomfortable take-it-or-leave-it situations, and if they don't approve the protocol as written, they lose the opportunity to run the trial and the funding that goes along with that.

It's unclear how much of a problem this possibility truly presents. IRB members insist that they examine protocols for multicenter trials as carefully as trials that originate within their own institutions, and they say they're not afraid to demand changes when necessary. Dr. Santana gives this example:

> *I remember one protocol that was submitted after already being activated at another hospital. The IRB felt very strongly that there was a flaw in the study design, and we said, "We will not approve this study, for these specific reasons. Go back to the cooperative-group committee and raise these concerns." Lo and behold, the problem was recognized and fixed, and the protocol came back to us. It's naive to assume that if it has been approved by other IRBs, it's flawless.*

Data Safety and Monitoring Boards

In addition to approving protocols, IRBs are charged with monitoring ongoing clinical trials. They review these trials annually to ensure that the protocol is being followed and that there's no excessive toxicity. In multicenter trials, however, especially in randomized Phase III trials, the NCI requires another level of oversight.

This is called the Data Safety and Monitoring Board (DSMB), also referred to as the Data Monitoring Committee (DMC). DSMBs are established at the level of the cooperative group. DSMB members are independent experts who are selected for their experience, objectivity, absence of conflicts of interest, and knowledge of clinical trials.

It's the job of the DSMB to examine the interim data emerging from an ongoing clinical trial and to determine whether the trial needs to be changed or terminated. For example, if the treatment under study seems to be causing too many adverse reactions, the DSMB might recommend that the dose be lowered or that the trial be ended. It can also recommend that the trial be ended if the experimental treatment is so effective that it would be unethical to continue giving some patients the standard treatment. In that case, all patients receiving the standard treatment would be given the opportunity to get the experimental treatment.

But DSMBs have their critics.[3] Unlike IRBs, DSMBs are not mandated by federal law and are not currently subject to federal regulation. Their critics note that although the responsibility for protecting subjects is assigned to the IRB, the exercise of that responsibility often falls to the DSMB, which is not accountable to and does not interact with any IRB. The critics reason that the DSMB's responsibilities and procedures ought to be codified. Although the NCI does have specific written policies governing the conduct of DSMBs, these policies might not have the force of law.

CHAPTER NINE

Financial Issues

THIS CHAPTER DISCUSSES SOME important monetary issues surrounding clinical trials. First there is some background on the rapidly increasing costs of drug development, of which clinical trials are a significant part. Next there is an examination of how these high costs (and disagreements about who will pay for them) can affect you. It can be difficult—but certainly not impossible—to get your insurance company to pay for the routine medical costs involved in clinical trials. In case your insurance company won't pay, this chapter presents some of the alternatives for funding medical care. The chapter concludes with an overview of agencies that can help you with the expenses associated with traveling to distant clinical trials.

The cost of drug development

Developing new drugs is almost unbelievably expensive. According to Ken Getz, president of CenterWatch, which publishes newsletters for the clinical trial industry, current estimates indicate that it will cost an average of $500 million dollars to develop each successful new drug entering research and development in 1998. For drugs that are coming to market now, the average development cost was $289 million. It takes twelve to fifteen years for a drug to make it through the pipeline from discovery, through preclinical development, through clinical trials, through the FDA approval process, to market. These figures include the amortized cost of unsuccessful drugs that never make it to market, but they do not include post-market costs, such as advertising and marketing.

Clinical trials are a big part of the high cost of drug development, and they're getting bigger. According to Getz, in the early 1990s the average new treatment was tested in roughly 32 to 36 distinct clinical studies of all phases. By the late 1990s that number had grown to about 68. Note that these figures are not inflated by the growing prevalence of multicenter trials. A study conducted at a dozen sites is considered a single one of those 68 trials. Getz explains:

> *Our research programs have gotten much more ambitious. The actual complexity of a protocol—the number of procedures that have to be conducted on a patient—has rapidly increased by as much as 30 to 40 percent in a particular phase of research. The actual number of patients enrolled in a trial has gone up dramatically. In the early '90s, the average number enrolled was around 2,400 or 2,500 for a single new drug application. Now that number is approaching 3,800 or 3,900. It's also costing more to find patients. We're competing for patients with more studies, so we're using more aggressive, expensive, and sophisticated advertising and promotion today to find these patients.*

But that's for the average new drug for all medical conditions. The costs for cancer drugs might be even higher, says Getz:

> *Cancer trials tend to have more complicated protocols and they do tend to be more expensive. You're asking the patient to do more in the trial—more lab tests, to keep a diary, and to undergo more experiences with a study drug.*

Payment for participation

Because participation in cancer clinical trials can sometimes be quite onerous for the patient, some cancer patients are actually compensated for their participation, and that adds to the cost of a clinical trial. Often the compensation is limited to reimbursement of out-of-pocket travel expenses, but occasionally, participants in cancer clinical trials will be paid up to $1,500.

Cash payments tend to be rare in NCI-sponsored trials, but are more common in trials sponsored by pharmaceutical companies. Payment tends to be higher in early-phase trials, which are more risky. Among trials that provide cash compensation, higher payments tend to be found in the more onerous trials—ones that require painful procedures or repeated visits. Don't expect to get rich participating in a clinical trial, however. Extremely high compensation would be considered unduly coercive and is thus unethical. (See Chapter 3, *Clinical Trial Ethics*.) The amount of cash compensation you stand to receive should play little or no role in your decision about whether to participate in a given trial.

Drug-company profits

Despite the high costs of drug development, you shouldn't feel too sorry for the pharmaceutical industry. That's because by almost any measure you care to examine, the pharmaceutical industry is the most profitable industry in the world.[1] According to a Philadelphia Inquirer investigation conducted in 1992, the median return on equity among Fortune 500 drug companies was 26 percent in 1991, almost twice the median for all Fortune 500 industries and first among 87 other industries. That figure had been above 20 percent since 1986 and above 15 percent since 1970, demonstrating that the industry remained robust throughout several boom-and-bust cycles in the overall economy. On the basis of return on assets, the pharmaceutical industry was first among 86 industries. And on the basis of return on sales, the pharmaceutical industry ranked third, just behind two utility groups. According to a more recent article in Fortune magazine, the industry's 15 to 16 percent annual growth rate looks "rock solid" for at least the next several years.[2] Clearly, the pharmaceutical industry is in the pink of health, even though drug development is enormously expensive.

Insurance coverage for trials

Whether you have traditional fee-for-service insurance, or you're one of the growing number of Americans who participate in a managed care plan such as an HMO, you might be worried that your medical coverage will not pay for your participation in a clinical trial. Unfortunately, your fears may be all too rational; most medical plans specifically exclude payments for experimental treatments. Among the lists of "exclusions" in their contracts is one that usually reads something like this:

> You will not receive benefits for the following: services and supplies which are experimental or investigational in nature, meaning any treatment, procedures, facility, equipment, drugs, drug usage, devices, or supplies not recognized as accepted medical procedure standards and any such items requiring federal or governmental agency approval not granted at the time services were rendered.

According to Ken Getz, the main reason that insurance providers remain reluctant to cover treatment in the context of clinical trials is that they're concerned that they may be liable if the study medication causes significant side effects:

> No one has figured out a way of limiting the liability of the insurance provider in the event that the patient has a long-term adverse reaction to a study medication. A lot of it is due to the pharmaceutical industry's inability to educate the insurance providers as well as they could. Insurance providers need to understand who is going to bear the burden of that cost in the event that the patient requires additional care after the study has ended. Normally the pharmaceutical industry does pay those costs, although industry can be rather elusive in accepting that commitment. There are times where a patient might have had a pre-existing condition that may or may not have been exacerbated by the study medication.

> There's an old adage in our industry: "Managed care and clinical research shall never mix." The greatest downside to that is that

we're not improving the access that patients have to an investiga-
tional treatment that could potentially save their lives. But
managed care organizations are starting to realize that if they
don't focus on demonstrating to the patient that they have their
best interests in mind, they're going to lose that membership.

There are recent indications that the message does seem to be getting through to the managed care industry. In February 1999, the
NIH reached an agreement with the American Association of
Health Plans (AAHP)—the trade group for the managed care industry—that calls for HMOs and other managed care organizations to
pay for the routine costs of members who enroll in NIH-sponsored
clinical trials for new drugs and medical procedures.[3]

Although this is very good news indeed, the agreement apparently
does have a number of significant shortcomings. First, although the
AAHP claims to represent about 1,000 managed care organizations,
not every HMO or PPO (preferred provider organization) is a member. Moreover, the agreement calls on AAHP merely to "encourage"
managed care plans to comply with the agreement, which does not
have the force of law. In addition, even managed care organizations
that choose to comply with the agreement are being asked only to
cover the routine costs of NIH-sponsored clinical trials, leaving in
the lurch patients who want to enroll in one of the many clinical
trials sponsored by pharmaceutical companies.

Don't despair if your insurance company or managed care provider
seems to exclude coverage for the clinical trial you want to participate in. There are strategies that may well help you get them to pay
for the non-experimental portion of your clinical trial, and as
you've already seen, the study's sponsor typically pays for the
experimental portion.

Jane H. Bick, PhD, offers this perspective:

I don't believe that insurance companies should pay for the cost
of research. I don't believe they should pay for data management

*or for the cost of investigational drugs. I do believe they should pay
routine medical costs that they would pay anyway. They should
not abandon a cancer patient who has the opportunity to go on a
study.*

Most clinical trials at most institutions employ someone who will
help you deal with your insurance company or managed care
provider. Ask the coordinator of your clinical trial if you can have
access to such a person. If this person is available as a resource, it's
a good idea to work with him from the beginning instead of after
problems arise. He will have knowledge of how the insurance
industry in general—and probably also your specific provider—
works and can often head off difficulties before they start. If you
don't have access to such a person, you can use the same strategies
they do in your negotiations for insurance coverage.

Gregory T. David, a nurse coordinator at the University of
California, San Francisco, and his colleague Robert L. Kuhn, a clinical research associate, point out that although they generally don't
have trouble getting insurance companies to cover the costs of standard care, it's sometimes a challenge to convince an HMO to cover
certain laboratory tests that must be performed outside the HMO's
facilities.

Mr. David says of a current study:

*This particular study is a combination of standard-care therapy
and experimental therapy. It's up to the insurance company to
understand that they're responsible for everything that's "standard
of care." They're not financially responsible for anything else. The
study picks up the costs of that. The problem is that much of the
"standard of care" stuff has to be done here, which is "out of
house" from their point of view. That's where the difficulty is in
getting insurance companies to go along. It usually just takes a little more time, a week or two weeks, to get them to play. It requires
careful documentation, careful communication between us.*

Mr. Kuhn notes:

The trial sponsors do not require us to have all these assessments—lab tests, radiology assessments, and so on—at our own institution. The HMOs generally want to do as much as they can in house because it's less expensive for them. They will authorize us to treat the patient here. The patients receive their chemotherapy here, and they'll have their periodic visits with our oncologist here, and sometimes because of necessity we will do lab work on the day of treatment. But follow-up tests to monitor blood count, liver function, adrenals, and things like that will be done at the HMO.

Negotiating where certain procedures are going to be performed works well if your insurance company seems as if it's going to be reasonable. Unfortunately, some are not. Jane H. Bick, who's on the board of the Atlanta-based organization CURE Childhood Cancer, points out that when dealing with insurance companies, discretion is often the better part of valor:

Sometimes clinical trials are not new drugs. They're new combinations of existing drugs. But the minute you say "clinical trial" or "investigational therapy," they say, "Sorry, we're not going to cover anything here." Therefore, many people are participating in clinical trials, and if it's not a brand new drug, their insurance companies don't know it. Never ever use the words "investigational drug" or "experimental" or "clinical trial" with your insurance company. It's like fanning the fire.

Under the old days of fee-for-service insurance, insurers never asked what drugs you were being given, what frequency, what dosage, whether you were an in-patient or an out-patient. They didn't ask for details; they just paid the bills. So people were participating in clinical trials without much objection from their insurance companies. Now, under managed care, payers want to know everything. Then they look at their little protocol sheets and

*see that this is not one of the approved protocols, and they deny
care.*

Lydia Cunningham Rising faced this dilemma when she was helping her ex-husband who, you will recall from Chapter 2, enrolled
in a clinical trial involving blood-brain barrier disruption. She
knew that each chemotherapy session would cost $10,000 and that
Joe would need several of them, and she wanted to find out in
advance whether their insurance company would cover it. She
planned to ask the insurance company directly, but the people running her trial advised against it. They believed that if she asked
straight out whether they covered blood-brain barrier disruption,
the insurance company would say, "What on earth is that?" and
deny the claim. Instead, the hospital billed the procedure as "intra-
arterial chemotherapy with brain tumor perfusion." Intra-arterial
chemotherapy was a common procedure, and the drugs they were
using were also standard. Only the delivery method was experimental. As it turned out, the insurance company didn't bat an eye,
but the Cunninghams spent an anxious three months—and ran up
a $30,000 bill—before they found out for sure that their insurance
company would pay.

Even if your insurance company or HMO explicitly denies care,
you still shouldn't give up, says Jane Bick:

> *It's so hard to fight the disease, and your family is in a state of
> shock. How can you fight your insurance company when you're
> fighting the disease? But you have to fight because it's about
> survival.*

> *If you want to enter a clinical trial for a medication that has
> already been approved for another condition, or at a different
> dosage, you can often invoke your state's "off-label" law. Not all
> states have an off-label law, but those that do permit physicians to
> prescribe at will any medication that's been approved for use in
> one situation. If this is the case, your insurance company may not
> need to know that you're participating in a clinical trial. You'll*

simply submit your bills for reimbursement just as you would for
any other medical treatment.

In her former capacity as managed care coordinator at Boston's Brigham and Women's Hospital, Maria A. Infantine-Harwood (currently vice president for product management at Boston Life Sciences, Inc.) often found herself negotiating with HMOs to cover some of the costs of clinical trials. "Treatments or medications already approved by the FDA would usually be covered by HMOs," she says.

But if your state doesn't have an off-label law, or if you want to enter a clinical trial for a treatment that has not yet been approved, you can employ other strategies. Even if the FDA has not approved a certain medication, you might be able to find evidence that your insurance company or HMO has paid a similar claim from another patient, possibly in a different state. If that's the case, you can use this evidence as leverage to encourage them to pay your claim. Ms. Harwood gives this example:

> *I remember one instance where there was a patient who wished*
> *to participate in a cancer clinical trial, and the HMO was denying*
> *treatment. I wondered what I could do to prove to them that this*
> *was something that had been used before and had been covered. I*
> *actually found a lawsuit that was won by a patient in California*
> *for the same treatment. I found enough documentation to prove to*
> *the HMO that this would really benefit the patient, and they*
> *should not deny it.*

Joyce Niblack recalls her experience as a clinical trial participant:

> *When you have a drug that's not approved for your diagnosis,*
> *the insurance company can say, "Well, it's experimental, and we're*
> *not going to pay for it." That was my experience with interferon in*
> *1989. Fortunately, there was quite a bit of literature on interferon,*
> *and the manufacturer provided me with abstracts of literature*
> *citations showing use in my condition. I also managed to get a*
> *printout of all the interferon claims that had been paid by the*

> same insurance company and a letter from my doctor explaining
> my need for this drug. I submitted a request for reconsideration
> and supported it by the thick stack of documents I had gathered,
> particularly pointing out that they had approved claims for this
> drug for others. They ended up paying for my treatment.

Sometimes even rational arguments do not have much influence within the often mysterious confines of health insurance companies. When that happens, Jane Bick advises:

> Go public. Insurance companies fear only two things: a court of
> law and the court of public opinion. And a lot of pressure can be
> brought to bear on insurance companies through the media and
> through attorneys. If they know that you've talked to attorneys
> and that you're talking to the media, all of a sudden they reconsid-
> er. There are attorneys who will take these cases either on
> contingency or for a small fee. Sometimes all it takes is one letter
> from a law office, and all of a sudden the insurance company says,
> "We'd better pay attention to this one."

As you no doubt have realized by now, some of the strategies suggested here are mutually contradictory. You can't conceal the fact that you're in a clinical trial from your insurance company while simultaneously negotiating with them on where to conduct certain tests. What works in one situation with one insurance company will not work with another. Seek expert advice on these matters whenever possible.

Legislative action

Of course, anyone with cancer realizes that it's ridiculous, maddening, and demeaning for a person facing a life-threatening illness to have to play these games with an insurance company in order to get coverage for a clinical trial.

And it's short-sighted on the part of the insurance companies and managed care organizations as well. The more rapidly treatments for cancer are developed, the more money they will save. New treatments are likely to be more effective and have fewer side effects than the old ones, requiring less medical care for those who receive them. Health insurance companies should be encouraging their members to investigate clinical trials instead of placing obstacles in their paths.

This argument often falls on deaf ears in the insurance industry. If the industry won't voluntarily cover the standard medical care associated with clinical trials, we'll all have to encourage our elected representatives to pass laws that will force the industry to do what's right. As of this writing, three states—Maryland, Rhode Island, and Georgia—have enacted laws mandating coverage for some kinds of clinical trials. Similar laws have been proposed in several other states and at the federal level as well.

Maryland's law is the most comprehensive. Passed in 1998, it requires insurers to pay "the cost of a medically necessary health-care service that is incurred as a result of the treatment being provided to the member for purposes of the clinical trial." It specifically excludes payments for the cost of the investigational drug or device or any costs involved in administering the clinical trial.

The law covers trials in phases I, II, III, and IV for people with cancer, but only phases II and III for people with other life-threatening diseases. To be covered, the trial must be approved by the National Institutes of Health or one of its cooperative groups, the FDA, or the federal Department of Veterans Affairs. The law also covers trials conducted by academic medical centers in Maryland. The law states that insurers must pay for patient costs incurred in trials for which "there is no clearly superior noninvestigational treatment alternative; and the available clinical or preclinical data provide a reasonable expectation that the treatment will be at least as effective as the noninvestigational alternative."

In Rhode Island, a similar law is restricted to Phase II and III clinical trials for cancer.

Jane Bick was instrumental in getting Georgia's law passed in 1998. This law requires health insurers (but not companies that self-insure their employees) to cover the routine medical costs for children enrolled in Phase II, III, and IV cancer trials:

> *It only covers children because we were told that was all we could expect to get passed in the '98 session. Georgia is a strong pro-business state, and it has a very active insurance lobby. They fight everything, and their mantra is, "If you pass this, it'll raise premiums, and many more small businesses in Georgia won't be able to insure their employees." That's simply not true, especially for cancer clinical trials. Insurers already pay routine medical costs for standard therapy. This bill was to prevent payer abandonment of kids in studies.*

Despite restricting the proposed bill to children with cancer, getting it passed was quite a challenge, says Bick. "It took blood, sweat, toil, and tears and a lot of hard work by a lot of people who really care about kids with cancer."

As a board member of CURE Children's Cancer, Bick managed to assemble a coalition of other cancer organizations to help push for the bill's passage. Among the people she recruited was Mo Thrash, a former CURE president who is also an experienced lobbyist with intimate knowledge of how things work in the Georgia legislature. Thrash (who had lost one of his children to leukemia twenty years previously) was able to get the ear of important legislators. He was also able to give valuable advice on encouraging public support for the bill, such as when to have people call their senators and representatives. Bick herself coordinated the strategic appearance of, as she puts it, "cute, bald-headed kids":

> *Legislators can't fix problems if they don't know the problems exist. I hate to talk in clichés, but one of the things we found was that squeaky wheels get greased. We had so many phone calls going into the Georgia legislature that legislative staff members were saying, "What is this bill? It must be an important one."*

Remarkably, the bill ended up passing unanimously in both houses of the Georgia legislature. It was named Callaway's Law in memory of Thrash's son.

At the federal level, broad access to clinical trials was an important part of a bill called the Patients' Bill of Rights Act of 1998, introduced by Senator Thomas A. Daschle (D-SD) in the Senate and by Congressman John Dingell (D-MI) in the House of Representatives. The bill would have required that any health insurer cover the "routine patient costs for items and services furnished in connection with participation" in a clinical trial for anyone who has "a life-threatening or serious illness for which no standard treatment is effective." The bill would have covered all phases of clinical trials as long as it was a trial approved by the National Institutes of Health or its cooperative groups, the Department of Veterans Affairs, or the Department of Defense.

Unfortunately, the bill never emerged from committee in the 105th Congress, but its supporters vowed to reintroduce it in the next Congress. Perhaps by the time you read this book, we will have comprehensive federal legislation guaranteeing patients access to clinical trials.

If such legislation has not yet passed, and if you believe health insurance providers should be required to cover the routine medical costs of patients enrolled in approved clinical trials, contact your state and federal representatives. All it would take is a short, polite letter, a phone call, or an email citing the importance of clinical trials and urging the representative to support appropriate legislation. If you're more ambitious, if you have specific legislative savvy, or if you're involved with a cancer society, you might want to follow Jane Bick's lead and help organize a broad-based coalition of organizations to lobby your state legislature—or the US Congress—for passage of a specific bill.

Paying to participate

Even if you don't have health insurance or you can't get your insurance company to pay for your participation in a clinical trial, you might still be able to participate, but you might have to pay for the routine medical costs yourself. If you're in that position, here are a few suggestions:

- If you have money saved for a rainy day, that day has come.

- You might be able to withdraw cash from retirement or pension accounts.

- Gain access to the equity in your home by taking out a second mortgage or a reverse mortgage.

- If you have life insurance, you may qualify for accelerated death benefits or a viatical settlement. In an accelerated death benefit, the insurance company pays you a percentage of the value of your policy before your death. Viatical settlements are cash lump sums given by investors to terminally ill people in exchange for the death benefits of their life insurance. For more information on these options, see the site *http://www.viaticalexpert.net*.

- Have your friends or co-workers organize a fundraiser to help you pay for your treatments.

- Try to interest local newspaper or television reporters in writing or broadcasting stories about your plight.

- Some organizations offer financial aid to people with cancer. For example, the Leukemia Society of America offers patients up to $750 per year in reimbursement for things such as travel, approved drugs, blood transfusions, and x-rays. LISA will reimburse expenses incurred only after you have applied for aid. Call (800) 955-4LISA. The National Children's Cancer Society, Inc., also provides some financial assistance. Call (800) 5-FAMILY.

- Check with your church or any fraternal organizations to which you belong; many of them maintain funds for members to use in emergencies.

This discussion has dealt with the typical situation in which a clinical trial's sponsor pays for any investigational treatment, and the patient or her insurance company pays for only the routine medical care associated with that treatment. In recent years, however, a small number of for-profit companies have sprung up in the US that charge people large sums of money for the privilege of participating in clinical trials.[4] Some of these companies have charged people with cancer as much as $30,000 to receive investigational treatments.

Although such practices have been defended as necessary for researchers who are unable to obtain research funding by other means, people with cancer should be exceedingly wary about pursuing fee-for-service research. The ethics of such a practice are questionable at best, and it would be difficult to separate serious and principled researchers who are merely using an innovative funding technique from snake-oil salesmen who are intent on exploiting you for their benefit.

Traveling for treatment

With the growth of multicenter trials and the success of NCI's Community Clinical Oncology Program (both of which are discussed in Chapter 8, *Administration of Clinical Trials*), fewer people with cancer are finding it necessary to travel long distances to participate in clinical trials. Nevertheless, you might find that the best clinical trial for your situation is many miles away.

Travel presents both financial and logistical problems for a person with cancer and his or her family. Fortunately, there are solutions to most of these problems.[5]

If you need to travel for a clinical trial, the first thing you should do is check with the people running the trial to see whether the trial itself will cover some or all of your travel expenses. This is a common practice, whether the trial is in your own city (in which case you might be able to get your taxi fare reimbursed) or somewhere far away. Dr. Richard Gams confirms this practice:

> *If our study required patients to make an additional trip that wouldn't help them particularly but is necessary to learn something about the drug, then often it's considered appropriate not only to pay for the test, but to reimburse the patient for travel expenses.*

Second, you should check your health insurance policy, which might cover some travel expenses. Some policies cover airfare but not lodging, others will pay a daily rate to reimburse you for food and lodging but won't pay for airfare, others will pay you for travel on a per-mile basis, and still others won't pay a dime. Also, make sure you know your insurance carrier's policy regarding emergency care when you're outside its service area. This can be a particular concern if you're enrolled in an HMO.

Air travel

If you need to travel by air to a clinical trial, a number of organizations can help, but some of them have certain restrictions, requiring, for example, that you be able to embark and disembark the plane without the airline's assistance. The best place to start your inquiries is Mercy Medical Airlift's National Patient Air Transport Helpline (NPATH), at (800) 296-1217.

Mercy Medical Airlift (MMA) coordinates three sectors of charitable air services in the US—the corporate aviation sector, the private aviation sector, and the commercial airline sector. MMA uses fixed-wing aircraft to help financially needy patients go to and from care centers for scheduled appointments, but it does not provide emergency transport. Mercy Medical Airlift can be contacted at (800) 296-1191.

The corporate aviation sector includes 750 corporations who are part of the Corporate Angel Network. Participating companies allow cancer patients to use empty seats on regularly scheduled corporate flights. You need not demonstrate financial hardship to use this service, and there's no limit to the number of trips you may take. Adult cancer patients may travel with a single companion, and children may be accompanied by two parents. Call (914) 328-1313 for more information.

The private aviation sector includes 4,500 pilots and 32 volunteer pilot organizations across the US who use their own time and aircraft to fly patients free-of-charge to care centers. These groups are part of the Air Care Alliance. Call (888) 662-6794 for more information.

In the past, some commercial airlines have occasionally offered special fares or even free tickets for people who must travel for medical care. Unfortunately, such programs are becoming increasingly rare. Contacting the airline directly through its reservations desk will generally prove unproductive, so it's best to work through MMA when pursuing this option.

Ground transportation

Some local offices of the American Cancer Society have networks of volunteers who will drive you to your treatment center. You can find a list of local ACS offices by phoning (800) ACS-2345, or on the web at *http://www.cancer.org/bottomdivisions.html*.

Lodging

Once you get to the city where you'll be receiving treatment, you'll face the problem of finding a place to stay. Often you'll be receiving treatment as an outpatient, perhaps for an extended period, and unless you're wealthy, four-star hotels are probably out of the question. It would be nice to find a place near the hospital where you and your family could stay at little or no cost, preferably one with kitchen and laundry facilities. Fortunately, there are a number of possibilities.

The ACS maintains Hope Lodges in many major cities that provide free housing on a first-come, first-serve basis for people being treated for cancer and their families. Hope Lodges have kitchen and laundry facilities. For information, phone (800) ACS-2345.

The National Association of Hospital Hospitality Houses maintains a list of facilities set up to provide free or low-cost housing to patients being treated at nearby hospitals or their families. The houses range in size from 6 to 64 rooms and typically have a common living area. Most have kitchens and laundry facilities as well. For information, phone (800) 542-9730.

The Ronald McDonald Houses sponsored by the McDonald's Corporation offer lodging to children and their families traveling for medical care. You might need to demonstrate financial hardship to be permitted to stay at some facilities. Others charge a nominal fee of $10 per night, which may be waived if you can demonstrate financial hardship. For information, phone (312) 836-7100.

The National Cancer Institute (NCI) offers meals and housing in its Children's Inn for patients under eighteen being treated at NCI. Family members can be accommodated on occasion. For information, phone (800) 4-CANCER.

Family members of people being treated at NCI are sometimes permitted to stay overnight in the patient's room. You should verify the availability of this option when making arrangements and again with the nurses on your floor.

Many hospitals make individual arrangements with nearby hotels for reduced rates for the families of patients. Check with the hospital's social worker or admitting desk for more information.

Additionally, some major medical centers, such as the Johns Hopkins Medical Institutions in Baltimore, maintain outpatient facilities for patients and their families.

Resources

This appendix gathers resources mentioned elsewhere in the book. Note that this is not meant to be an exhaustive list of resources related to cancer. There are dozens of organizations, hundreds of books, and probably thousands of Internet sites devoted to all aspects of cancer research and cancer treatment. This is a highly selective list of resources related to cancer clinical trials.

Organizations

The National Cancer Institute (NCI) is the largest of the seventeen institutes that compose the National Institutes of Health (NIH), which in turn is part of the Department of Health and Human Services. Located in Bethesda, Maryland, the NCI is the nation's premier center for cancer research. You'll find a great deal of information about cancer and the NCI on its main web page at *http://www.nci.nih.gov/*. NCI operates a valuable toll-free telephone number called the Cancer Information Service at (800) 4-CANCER. At that number, you can order books, pamphlets, and videos on many cancer-related subjects, and you can request a list of all clinical trials for your condition. NCI also operates the Physicians Data Query (PDQ) web site (discussed in the section on Internet sites later in this appendix).

Office for Protection from Research Risks (OPRR)

Division of Human Subject Protections
National Institutes of Health
6100 Executive Blvd., Ste. 3B01 (MSC 7507)
Rockville, MD 20892-7507
(301) 496-7041
(301) 402-0527 (fax)
http://www.nih.gov:80/grants/oprr/oprr.htm
OPRR is charged with enforcing federal regulations regarding clinical trials.

Food and Drug Administration (FDA)

http://www.fda.gov/
If you have difficulties with a pharmaceutical company's conduct of a clinical trial, you can seek a resolution with the FDA's Center for Drug Evaluation and Research.

Center for Drug Evaluation and Research

http://www.fda.gov/cder/
In particular, you might want to contact James C. Morrison, the CDER Ombudsman.

James C. Morrison, CDER Ombudsman (HFD-1)

5600 Fishers Lane
Rockville, MD 20857
(301) 594-5443
(301) 827-4312 (fax)
morrisonj@cder.fda.gov
http://www.fda.gov/cder/ombud.htm

FDA's Consumer Complaint Coordinators

http://www.fda.gov/opacom/backgrounders/problem.html.
You'll find a complete list of phone numbers for each state at this site.

American Cancer Society
(800) ACS-2345
http://www.cancer.org/
The nation's premier cancer charity. Through its 3,400 local offices, the ACS provides support groups and many other services for people with cancer.

Books

Bazell, Robert. *Her-2: The Making of Herceptin, a Revolutionary Treatment for Breast Cancer.* New York: Random House, 1998. NBC science correspondent Robert Bazell has written a gripping account of the development of Herceptin, including detailed descriptions of the clinical trials and many of the courageous participants.

Dorland, W. A. Newman, ed. *Dorland's Illustrated Medical Dictionary.* Troy, MO: W. B. Saunders Co., 1994. Valuable technical information.

Harrington, Anne, editor. *The Placebo Effect: An Interdisciplinary Exploration.* Cambridge: Harvard University Press, 1997. A thorough discussion of the placebo effect.

Jones, James H. *Bad Blood: The Tuskegee Syphilis Experiment.* New York: Free Press, 1993. This is the second edition of the definitive book on the Tuskegee experiment.

Lerner, Michael. *Choices in Healing: Integrating the Best of Conventional and Complementary Approaches to Cancer.* Cambridge: MIT Press, 1994. This book will give you a thorough overview of integrating conventional and complementary approaches to cancer treatments. It's also available online, in its entirety, at *http://www.commonweal.org/choicescontents.html.*

Lifton, Robert Jay. *The Nazi Doctors: Medical Killing and the Psychology of Genocide.* New York: Basic Books, 1986. This book contains a detailed discussion of the Nazi medical experiments and the context in which they occurred.

Murphy, Gerald P., MD, Lois B. Morris, and Dianne Lange. *Informed Decisions: The Complete Book of Cancer Diagnosis, Treatment, and Recovery*. New York: Viking Penguin Books, 1997. Sponsored by the American Cancer Society, *Informed Decisions* is an excellent source of information on specific cancers, their standard treatments, and their likely outcomes.

Schine, Gary, with Ellen Berlinsky. *Cancer Cure: How To Find And Get The Best There Is* (formerly titled *If the President Had Cancer...*). New York: Kensington Books, 1994. This book will help you research your medical condition and make informed decisions on your care.

Shapiro, Arthur K., and Elaine Shapiro. *The Powerful Placebo: From Ancient Priest to Modern Physician*. Baltimore: Johns Hopkins University Press, 1997. A thorough discussion of the placebo effect.

Stedman, Thomas Lathrop. *Stedman's Medical Dictionary*. Baltimore: Lippincott Williams & Wilkins, 1995. Valuable technical information.

Thomas, Clayton L., editor. *Taber's Cyclopedic Medical Dictionary*. Philadelphia: F.A. Davis Co., 1997. Valuable technical information.

Vanderpool, Harold Y., editor. *The Ethics of Research Involving Human Subjects: Facing the 21st Century*. Frederick, Maryland: University Publishing Group, Inc., 1996. This book contains chapters by eighteen renowned experts on the ethics of clinical trials.

Internet resources

Association of Cancer Online Resources
http://www.medinfo.org/
The best collection of email discussion lists related to cancer.

CancerGuide

http://www.cancerguide.org/

Maintained by cancer survivor Steve Dunn. CancerGuide contains basic information about cancer, links that will help you research your condition, information on clinical trials, and inspirational patient stories.

The CenterWatch Clinical Trials Listing Service

http://www.centerwatch.com

A searchable database of 7,500 current clinical trials in all areas of medicine, including cancer.

Code of Federal Regulations, Title 45, Part 46, "Protection of Human Subjects"

http://www.med.umich.edu/irbmed/FederalDocuments/hhs/HHS45-CFR46.html

The full text of the regulations that govern all clinical trials in the US.

EurekAlert

http://www.eurekalert.org/

Searchable collections of cancer-related news releases from academic institutions.

Excite Newstracker

http://nt.excite.com/

Find current newspaper and magazine articles on any topic.

Internet Grateful Med

http://igm.nlm.nih.gov/

One way to access Medline, an index of the entire world's medical literature from 1966 to the present.

Newswise

http://www.newswise.com/

See "EurekAlert."

Patient Advocacy Home Page
http://uhec.udmercy.edu/picct/risinglo.htm
Maintained by Lydia Cunningham Rising. Along with several interesting articles—including one on "How to Talk (Back) to Your Doctor"—the site gives you the opportunity to complete a survey on your experiences with and attitude toward cancer clinical trials.

Physicians Data Query (PDQ)
http://cancertrials.nci.nih.gov/
The single best way to find cancer clinical trials. Maintained by NCI and PDQ, it is an easily searchable registry of more than 1,500 clinical trials in cancer.

PubMed
http://www4.ncbi.nlm.nih.gov/PubMed/
Another way to access Medline.

WebMD
http://my.webmd.com
A collection of communities of people with serious health concerns. Several of these communities relate to specific types of cancer.

Usenet Newsgroups Related to Cancer
- alt.support.cancer
- alt.support.cancer.breast
- alt.support.cancer.prostate
- alt.support.cancer.testicular
- sci.med.diseases.cancer

Research Services
The Health Resource, Inc.
933 Faulkner Street
Conway, AR 72032
(501) 329-5272
(800) 949-0090
http://thehealthresource.com/

MEDcetera, Inc.
(800) 748-6866
pgeyer@netropolis.net
http://www.netropolis.net/pgeyer/

Schine On-Line Services
39 Brenton Avenue
Providence, RI 02906
(401) 751-0120
(800) 346-3287
schine@findcure.com
http://www.findcure.com/

Help with travel and lodging

ACS Hope Lodges
(800) ACS-2345

Air Care Alliance
(888) 662-6794

Corporate Angel Network
(914) 328-1313

National Association of Hospital Hospitality Houses
(800) 542-9730

National Patient Air Transport Helpline (NPATH)
(800) 296-1217

Ronald McDonald Houses
(312) 836-7100

Critical Public Documents

The Nuremberg Code

The Nuremberg Code was developed in the aftermath of World War II and reads as follows:[1]

The great weight of the evidence before us is to the effect that certain types of medical experiments on human beings, when kept within reasonably well-defined bounds, conform to the ethics of the medical profession generally. The protagonists of the practice of human experimentation justify their views on the basis that such experiments yield results for the good of society that are unprocurable by other methods or means of study. All agree, however, that certain basic principles must be observed in order to satisfy moral, ethical and legal concepts:

1. The voluntary consent of the human subject is absolutely essential.

    This means that the person involved should have legal capacity to give consent; should be so situated as to be able to exercise free power of choice, without the intervention of any element of force, fraud, deceit, duress, overreaching, or other ulterior form of constraint or coercion; and should have sufficient knowledge and comprehension of the elements of the subject matter involved as to enable him to make an understanding and enlightened decision. This latter element requires that before the acceptance of an affirmative decision by the experimental subject, there should be made known to him the nature, duration, and purpose of the experiment; the method and means by which it is to be conducted; all inconveniences and hazards reasonably to be expected; and the effects upon his health or person that may possibly come from his participation in the experiment.

The duty and responsibility for ascertaining the quality of the consent rests upon each individual who initiates, directs, or engages in the experiment. It is a personal duty and responsibility that may not be delegated to another with impunity.

2. The experiment should be such as to yield fruitful results for the good of society, unprocurable by other methods or means of study and not random and unnecessary in nature.

3. The experiment should be so designed and based on the results of animal experimentation and a knowledge of the natural history of the disease or other problems under study that the anticipated results will justify the performance of the experiment.

4. The experiment should be so conducted as to avoid all unnecessary physical and mental suffering and injury.

5. No experiment should be conducted where there is an *a priori* reason to believe that death or disabling injury will occur; except perhaps, in those experiments where the experimental physicians also serve as subjects.

6. The degree of risk to be taken should never exceed that determined by the humanitarian importance of the problem to be solved by the experiment. Proper preparations should be made and adequate facilities provided to protect the experimental subject against even remote possibilities of injury, disability, or death.

7. The experiment should be conducted only by scientifically qualified persons. The highest degree of skill and care should be required through all stages of the experiment of those who conduct or engage in the experiment.

8. During the course of the experiment, the human subject should be at liberty to bring the experiment to an end if he has reached the physical or mental state where continuation of the experiment seems to him to be impossible.

9. During the course of the experiment, the scientist in charge must be prepared to terminate the experiment at any stage, if he has probable cause to believe in the exercise of the good faith, superior skill, and careful judgment required of him that a continuation of the experiment is likely to result in injury, disability, or death to the experimental subject.

The Belmont Report

The Belmont Report is a critical public document regarding research ethics.[2] The document's notes, indicated by letters, can be found at the end of the document.

Ethical Principles and Guidelines for the Protection of Human Subjects of Research

The National Commission for the Protection of Human Subjects of Biomedical and Behavioral Research

April 18, 1979

Scientific research has produced substantial social benefits. It has also posed some troubling ethical questions. Public attention was drawn to these questions by reported abuses of human subjects in biomedical experiments, especially during the Second World War. During the Nuremberg War Crime Trials, the Nuremberg Code was drafted as a set of standards for judging physicians and scientists who had conducted biomedical experiments on concentration camp prisoners. This code became the prototype of many later codes[a] intended to assure that research involving human subjects would be carried out in an ethical manner.

The codes consist of rules, some general, others specific, that guide the investigators or the reviewers of research in their work. Such rules often are inadequate to cover complex situations; at times they come into conflict, and they are frequently difficult to interpret or apply. Broader ethical principles will provide a basis on which specific rules may be formulated, criticized, and interpreted.

Three principles, or general prescriptive judgments, that are relevant to research involving human subjects are identified in this statement. Other principles may also be relevant. These three are comprehensive, however, and are stated at a level of generalization that should assist scientists, subjects, reviewers, and interested citizens to understand the ethical issues inherent in research involving human subjects. These principles cannot always be applied so as to resolve beyond dispute particular ethical problems. The objective is to provide an analytical framework that will guide the resolution of ethical problems arising from research involving human subjects.

This statement consists of a distinction between research and practice, a discussion of the three basic ethical principles, and remarks about the application of these principles.

A. Boundaries between practice and research

It is important to distinguish between biomedical and behavioral research, on the one hand, and the practice of accepted therapy on the other, in order to know what activities ought to undergo review for the protection of human subjects of research. The distinction between research and practice is blurred partly because both often occur together (as in research designed to evaluate a therapy) and partly because notable departures from standard practice are often called "experimental" when the terms "experimental" and "research" are not carefully defined.

For the most part, the term "practice" refers to interventions that are designed solely to enhance the well-being of an individual patient or client and that have a reasonable expectation of success. The purpose of medical or behavioral practice is to provide diagnosis, preventive treatment, or therapy to particular individuals.[b] By contrast, the term "research" designates an activity designed to test a hypothesis, permit conclusions to be drawn, and thereby to develop or contribute to generalizable knowledge (expressed, for example, in theories, principles, and statements of relationships). Research is usually described in a formal protocol that sets forth an objective and a set of procedures designed to reach that objective.

When a clinician departs in a significant way from standard or accepted practice, the innovation does not, in and of itself, constitute research. The fact that a procedure is "experimental," in the sense of new, untested, or different, does not automatically place it in the category of research. Radically new procedures of this description should, however, be made the object of formal research at an early stage in order to determine whether they are safe and effective. Thus, it is the responsibility of medical practice committees, for example, to insist that a major innovation be incorporated into a formal research project.[c]

Research and practice may be carried on together when research is designed to evaluate the safety and efficacy of a therapy. This need not cause any confusion regarding whether or not the activity requires review; the general rule is that if there is any element of research in an activity, that activity should undergo review for the protection of human subjects.

B. Basic ethical principles

The expression "basic ethical principles" refers to those general judgments that serve as a basic justification for the many particular ethical prescriptions and evaluations of human actions. Three basic principles, among those generally accepted in our cultural tradition, are particularly relevant to the ethics of research involving human subjects: the principles of respect for persons, beneficence, and justice.

1. Respect for Persons
Respect for persons incorporates at least two ethical convictions: first, that individuals should be treated as autonomous agents, and second, that persons with diminished autonomy are entitled to

protection. The principle of respect for persons thus divides into two separate moral requirements: the requirement to acknowledge autonomy and the requirement to protect those with diminished autonomy.

An autonomous person is an individual capable of deliberation about personal goals and of acting under the direction of such deliberation. To respect autonomy is to give weight to autonomous persons' considered opinions and choices while refraining from obstructing their actions unless they are clearly detrimental to others. To show lack of respect for an autonomous agent is to repudiate that person's considered judgments, to deny an individual the freedom to act on those considered judgments, or to withhold information necessary to make a considered judgment, when there are no compelling reasons to do so.

However, not every human being is capable of self-determination. The capacity for self-determination matures during an individual's life, and some individuals lose this capacity wholly or in part because of illness, mental disability, or circumstances that severely restrict liberty. Respect for the immature and the incapacitated may require protecting them as they mature or while they are incapacitated.

Some persons are in need of extensive protection, even to the point of excluding them from activities that may harm them; other persons require little protection beyond making sure they undertake activities freely and with awareness of possible adverse consequences. The extent of protection afforded should depend upon the risk of harm and the likelihood of benefit. The judgment that any individual lacks autonomy should be periodically reevaluated and will vary in different situations.

In most cases of research involving human subjects, respect for persons demands that subjects enter into the research voluntarily and with adequate information. In some situations, however, application of the principle is not obvious. The involvement of prisoners as subjects of research provides an instructive example. On the one hand, it would seem that the principle of respect for persons requires that prisoners not be deprived of the opportunity to volunteer for research. On the other hand, under prison conditions they may be subtly coerced or unduly influenced to engage in research activities for which they would not otherwise volunteer. Respect for persons would then dictate that prisoners be protected. Whether to allow prisoners to "volunteer" or to "protect" them presents a dilemma. Respecting persons, in most hard cases, is often a matter of balancing competing claims urged by the principle of respect itself.

2. Beneficence

Persons are treated in an ethical manner not only by respecting their decisions and protecting them from harm, but also by making efforts to secure their well-being. Such treatment falls under the principle of beneficence. The term "beneficence" is often understood to cover acts of kindness or charity that go beyond strict obligation. In this document, beneficence is understood in a stronger sense, as an obligation. Two general rules have been formulated as complementary expressions of beneficent actions in this sense: (1) do not harm and (2) maximize possible benefits and minimize possible harms.

The Hippocratic maxim "do no harm" has long been a fundamental principle of medical ethics. Claude Bernard extended it to the realm of research, saying that one should not injure one person regardless of the benefits that might come to others. However, even avoiding harm requires learning what is harmful; and in the process of obtaining this information, persons may be exposed to risk of harm. Further, the Hippocratic Oath requires physicians to benefit their patients "according to their best judgment." Learning what will in fact benefit may require exposing persons to risk. The problem posed by these imperatives is to decide when it is justifiable to seek certain benefits despite the risks involved and when the benefits should be foregone because of the risks.

The obligations of beneficence affect both individual investigators and society at large because they extend both to particular research projects and to the entire enterprise of research. In the case of particular projects, investigators and members of their institutions are obliged to give forethought to the maximization of benefits and the reduction of risk that might occur from the research investigation. In the case of scientific research in general, members of the larger society are obliged to recognize the longer term benefits and risks that may result from the improvement of knowledge and from the development of novel medical, psychotherapeutic, and social procedures.

The principle of beneficence often occupies a well-defined justifying role in many areas of research involving human subjects. An example is found in research involving children. Effective ways of treating childhood diseases and fostering healthy development are benefits that serve to justify research involving children—even when individual research subjects are not direct beneficiaries. Research also makes it possible to avoid the harm that may result from the application of previously accepted routine practices that on closer investigation turn out to be dangerous. But the role of the principle of beneficence is not always so unambiguous. A difficult ethical problem remains, for example, about research that presents more than minimal risk without immediate prospect of direct benefit to the children involved. Some have argued that such research is inadmissible, whereas others have pointed out that this limit would rule out much research promising great benefit to children in the future. Here again, as with all hard cases, the different claims covered by the principle of beneficence may come into conflict and force difficult choices.

3. Justice
Who ought to receive the benefits of research and bear its burdens? This is a question of justice, in the sense of "fairness in distribution" or "what is deserved." An injustice occurs when some benefit to which a person is entitled is denied without good reason or when some burden is imposed unduly. Another way of conceiving the

principle of justice is that equals ought to be treated equally. However, this statement requires explication. Who is equal and who is unequal? What considerations justify departure from equal distribution? Almost all commentators allow that distinctions based on experience, age, deprivation, competence, merit, and position do sometimes constitute criteria justifying differential treatment for certain purposes. It is necessary, then, to explain in what respects people should be treated equally. There are several widely accepted formulations of just ways to distribute burdens and benefits. Each formulation mentions some relevant property on the basis of which burdens and benefits should be distributed. These formulations are (1) to each person an equal share, (2) to each person according to individual need, (3) to each person according to individual effort, (4) to each person according to societal contribution, and (5) to each person according to merit.

Questions of justice have long been associated with social practices such as punishment, taxation, and political representation. Until recently these questions have not generally been associated with scientific research. However, they are foreshadowed even in the earliest reflections on the ethics of research involving human subjects. For example, during the 19th and early 20th centuries, the burdens of serving as research subjects fell largely upon poor ward patients, whereas the benefits of improved medical care flowed primarily to private patients. Subsequently, the exploitation of unwilling prisoners as research subjects in Nazi concentration camps was condemned as a particularly flagrant injustice. In this country, in the 1940s, the Tuskegee syphilis study used disadvantaged, rural black men to study the untreated course of a disease that is by no means confined to that population. These subjects were deprived of demonstrably effective treatment in order not to interrupt the project, long after such treatment became generally available.

Against this historical background, it can be seen how conceptions of justice are relevant to research involving human subjects. For example, the selection of research subjects needs to be scrutinized in order to determine whether some classes (e.g., welfare patients, particular racial and ethnic minorities, or persons confined to institutions) are being systematically selected simply because of their easy availability, their compromised position, or their manipulability, rather than for reasons directly related to the problem being studied. Finally, whenever research supported by public funds leads to the development of therapeutic devices and procedures, justice demands both that these not provide advantages only to those who can afford them and that such research should not unduly involve persons from groups unlikely to be among the beneficiaries of subsequent applications of the research.

C. Applications

Applications of the general principles to the conduct of research leads to consideration of the following requirements: informed consent, risk/benefit assessment, and the selection of subjects of research.

1. Informed Consent

Respect for persons requires that subjects, to the degree that they are capable, be given the opportunity to choose what shall or shall not happen to them. This opportunity is provided when adequate standards for informed consent are satisfied.

Although the importance of informed consent is unquestioned, controversy prevails over the nature and possibility of an informed consent. Nonetheless, there is widespread agreement that the consent process can be analyzed as containing three elements: information, comprehension, and voluntariness.

Information. Most codes of research establish specific items for disclosure intended to assure that subjects are given sufficient information. These items generally include the research procedure, their purposes, risks, and anticipated benefits, alternative procedures (where therapy is involved), and a statement offering the subject the opportunity to ask questions and to withdraw at any time from the research. Additional items have been proposed, including how subjects are selected, the person responsible for the research, and so on.

However, a simple listing of items does not answer the question of what the standard should be for judging how much and what sort of information should be provided. One standard frequently invoked in medical practice, namely the information commonly provided by practitioners in the field or in the locale, is inadequate because research takes place precisely when a common understanding does not exist. Another standard, currently popular in malpractice law, requires the practitioner to reveal the information that reasonable persons would wish to know in order to make a decision regarding their care. This, too, seems insufficient because the research subject, being in essence a volunteer, may wish to know considerably more about risks gratuitously undertaken than do patients who deliver themselves into the hand of a clinician for needed care. It may be that a standard of "the reasonable volunteer" should be proposed: the extent and nature of information should be such that persons, knowing that the procedure is neither necessary for their care nor perhaps fully understood, can decide whether they wish to participate in the furthering of knowledge. Even when some direct benefit to them is anticipated, the subjects should understand clearly the range of risk and the voluntary nature of participation.

A special problem of consent arises where informing subjects of some pertinent aspect of the research is likely to impair the validity of the research. In many cases, it is sufficient to indicate to subjects that they are being invited to participate in research of which some features will not be revealed until the research is concluded. In all cases of research involving incomplete disclosure, such research is justified only if it is clear that (1) incomplete disclosure is truly necessary to accomplish the goals of the research, (2) there are no undisclosed risks to subjects that are more than minimal, and (3) there is an adequate plan for debriefing subjects, when appropriate, and for dissemination of research results to them. Information about risks should never be withheld for the purpose of eliciting the cooperation of subjects, and truthful answers should always be given to direct questions about the research. Care should be taken to distinguish cases in which disclosure would destroy or invalidate the research from cases in which disclosure would simply inconvenience the investigator.

Comprehension. The manner and context in which information is conveyed is as important as the information itself. For example, presenting information in a disorganized and rapid fashion, allowing too little time for consideration, or curtailing opportunities for questioning all may adversely affect a subject's ability to make an informed choice.

Because the subject's ability to understand is a function of intelligence, rationality, maturity, and language, it is necessary to adapt the presentation of the information to the subject's capacities. Investigators are responsible for ascertaining that the subject has comprehended the information. Although there is always an obligation to ascertain that the information about risk to subjects is complete and adequately comprehended, when the risks are more serious, that obligation increases. On occasion, it may be suitable to give some oral or written tests of comprehension.

Special provisions may need to be made when comprehension is severely limited, for example, by conditions of immaturity or mental disability. Each class of subjects that one might consider as incompetent (e.g., infants and young children, mentally disabled patients, the terminally ill, and the comatose) should be considered on its own terms. Even for these persons, however, respect requires giving them the opportunity to choose to the extent they are able whether or not to participate in research. The objections of these subjects to involvement should be honored, unless the research entails providing them a therapy unavailable elsewhere. Respect for persons also requires seeking the permission of other parties in order to protect the subjects from harm. Such persons are thus respected both by acknowledging their own wishes and by the use of third parties to protect them from harm.

The third parties chosen should be those who are most likely to understand the incompetent subject's situation and to act in that person's best interest. The person authorized to act on behalf of the subject should be given an opportunity to observe the research as it proceeds in order to be able to withdraw the subject from the research, if such action appears in the subject's best interest.

Voluntariness. An agreement to participate in research constitutes a valid consent only if voluntarily given. This element of informed consent requires conditions free of coercion and undue influence. Coercion occurs when an overt threat of harm is intentionally presented by one person to another in order to obtain compliance. Undue influence, by contrast, occurs through an offer of an excessive, unwarranted, inappropriate, or improper reward or other overture in order to obtain compliance. Also, inducements that would ordinarily be acceptable may become undue influences if the subject is especially vulnerable.

Unjustifiable pressures usually occur when persons in positions of authority or commanding influence—especially where possible sanctions are involved—urge a course of action for a subject. A continuum of such influencing factors exists, however, and it is impossible to state precisely where justifiable persuasion ends and undue influence begins. But undue influence would include actions such as manipulating a person's choice through the controlling influence of a close relative and threatening to withdraw health services to which an individual would otherwise be entitled.

2. Assessment of Risks and Benefits

The assessment of risks and benefits requires a careful array of relevant data, including, in some cases, alternative ways of obtaining the benefits sought in the research. Thus, the assessment presents both an opportunity and a responsibility to gather systematic and comprehensive information about proposed research. For the investigator, it is a means to examine whether the proposed research is properly designed. For a review committee, it is a method for determining whether the risks that will be presented to subjects are justified. For prospective subjects, the assessment will assist the determination whether or not to participate.

The Nature and Scope of Risks and Benefits. The requirement that research be justified on the basis of a favorable risk/benefit assessment bears a close relation to the principle of beneficence, just as the moral requirement that informed consent be obtained is derived primarily from the principle of respect for persons. The term "risk" refers to a possibility that harm may occur. However, when expressions such as "small risk" or "high risk" are used, they usually refer (often ambiguously) both to the chance (probability) of experiencing a harm and the severity (magnitude) of the envisioned harm.

The term "benefit" is used in the research context to refer to something of positive value related to health or welfare. Unlike "risk," "benefit" is not a term that expresses probabilities. Risk is properly contrasted to probability of benefits, and benefits are properly contrasted with harms rather than risks of harm. Accordingly, so-called risk benefit assessments are concerned with the probabilities and magnitudes of possible harms and anticipated benefits. Many kinds of possible harms and benefits need to be taken into account. There are, for example, risks of psychological harm, physical harm, legal harm, social harm, and economic harm and the corresponding benefits. Although the most likely types of harms to research subjects are those of psychological or physical pain or injury, other possible kinds should not be overlooked.

Risks and benefits of research may affect the individual subjects, the families of the individual subjects, and society at large (or special groups of subjects in society). Previous codes and federal regulations have required that risks to subjects be outweighed by the sum of both the anticipated benefit to the subject, if any, and the anticipated benefit to society in the form of knowledge to be gained from the research. In balancing these different elements, the risks and benefits affecting the immediate research subject will normally carry special weight. On the other hand, interests other than those of the subject may on some occasions be sufficient by themselves to justify the risks involved in the research, so long as the subjects' rights have been protected. Beneficence thus requires that we protect against risk of harm to subjects and also that we be concerned about the loss of the substantial benefits that might be gained from research.

The Systematic Assessment of Risks and Benefits. It is commonly said that benefits and risks must be "balanced" and shown to be "in a favorable ratio." The metaphorical character of these terms draws attention to the difficulty of making precise judgments. Only on rare occasions will quantitative techniques be available for the scrutiny of research protocols. However, the idea of systematic, nonarbitrary analysis of risks and benefits should be emulated insofar as possible. This ideal requires those making decisions about the justifiability of research to be thorough in the accumulation and assessment of information about all aspects of the research and to consider alternatives systematically. This procedure renders the assessment of research more rigorous and precise, while making communication between review board members and investigators less subject to misinterpretation, misinformation, and conflicting judgments. Thus, there should first be a determination of the validity of the presuppositions of the research; then the nature, probability, and magnitude of risk should be distinguished with as much clarity as possible. The method of ascertaining risks should be explicit, especially where there is no alternative to the use of such vague categories as small or slight risk. It should also be determined whether an investigator's estimates of the probability of harm or benefits are reasonable, as judged by known facts or other available studies.

Finally, assessment of the justifiability of research should reflect at least the following considerations: (1) Brutal or inhumane treatment of human subjects is never morally justified. (2) Risks should be reduced to those necessary to achieve the research objective. It should be determined whether it is in fact necessary to use human subjects at all. Risk can perhaps never be entirely eliminated, but it can often be reduced by careful attention to alternative procedures. (3) When research involves significant risk of serious impairment, review committees should be extraordinarily insistent on the justification of the risk (looking usually to the likelihood of benefit to the subject or, in some rare cases, to the manifest voluntariness of the participation). (4) When vulnerable populations are involved in research, the appropriateness of involving them should itself be demonstrated. A number of variables go into such judgments, including the nature and degree of risk, the condition of the particular population involved, and the nature and level of the anticipated benefits. (5) Relevant risks and benefits must be thoroughly arrayed in documents and procedures used in the informed consent process.

3. Selection of Subjects

Just as the principle of respect for persons finds expression in the requirements for consent and the principle of beneficence in risk and benefit assessment, the principle of justice gives rise to moral requirements that there be fair procedures and outcomes in the selection of research subjects.

Justice is relevant to the selection of subjects of research at two levels: the social and the individual. Individual justice in the selection of subjects would require that researchers exhibit fairness; thus, they should not offer potentially beneficial research only to some patients who are in their favor or select only "undesirable" persons for risky research. Social justice requires that distinction be drawn between classes of subjects that ought, and ought not, to participate in any particular kind of research, based on the ability of members of that class to bear burdens and on the appropriateness of placing further burdens on already burdened persons. Thus, it can be considered a matter of social justice that there is an order of preference in the selection of classes of subjects (e.g., adults before children) and that some classes of potential subjects (e.g., the institutionalized mentally infirm or prisoners) may be involved as research subjects, if at all, only on certain conditions.

Injustice may appear in the selection of subjects, even if individual subjects are selected fairly by investigators and treated fairly in the course of research. Thus injustice arises from social, racial, sexual, and cultural biases institutionalized in society. Thus, even if individual researchers are treating their research subjects fairly, and even if IRBs are taking care to assure that subjects are selected fairly within a particular institution, unjust social patterns may nevertheless appear in the overall distribution of the burdens and benefits of research. Although individual institutions or investigators may not be able to resolve a problem that is pervasive in their social setting, they can consider distributive justice in selecting research subjects.

Some populations, especially institutionalized ones, are already burdened in many ways by their infirmities and environments. When research is proposed that involves risks and does not include a therapeutic component, other less burdened classes of persons should be called upon first to accept these risks of research, except where the research is directly related to the specific conditions of the class involved. Also, even though public funds for research may often flow in the same directions as public funds for healthcare, it seems unfair that populations dependent on public healthcare constitute a pool of preferred research subjects if more advantaged populations are likely to be the recipients of the benefits.

One special instance of injustice results from the involvement of vulnerable subjects. Certain groups, such as racial minorities, the economically disadvantaged, the very sick, and the institutionalized, may continually be sought as research subjects, owing to their ready availability in settings where research is conducted. Given their dependent status and their frequently compromised capacity for free consent, they should be protected against the danger of being involved in research solely for administrative convenience or because they are easy to manipulate as a result of their illness or socioeconomic condition.

The Belmont Report notes

a. Since 1945, various codes for the proper and responsible conduct of human experimentation in medical research have been adopted by different organizations. The best known of these codes are the Nuremberg Code of 1947, the Helsinki Declaration of 1964 (revised in 1975), and the 1971 Guidelines (codified into Federal Regulations in 1974) issued by the US Department of Health, Education, and Welfare. Codes for the conduct of social and behavioral research have also been adopted, the best known being that of the American Psychological Association, published in 1973.

b. Although practice usually involves interventions designed solely to enhance the well-being of a particular individual, interventions are sometimes applied to one individual for the enhancement of the well-being of another (e.g., blood donation, skin grafts, organ transplants), or an intervention might have the dual purpose of enhancing the well-being of a particular individual, and, at the same time, providing some benefit to others (e.g., vaccination, which protects both the person who is vaccinated and society generally). The fact that some forms of practice have elements other than immediate benefit to the individual receiving an intervention, however, should not confuse the general distinction between research and practice. Even when a procedure applied in practice might benefit some other person, it remains an intervention designed to enhance the well-being of a particular individual or groups of individuals; thus, it is practice and need not be reviewed as research.

c. Because the problems related to social experimentation might differ substantially from those of biomedical and behavioral research, the Commission specifically declines to make any policy determination regarding such research at this time. Rather, the Commission believes that the problem ought to be addressed by one of its successor bodies.

Notes

Chapter 1: *Overview of Clinical Trials*

1. Although this 5 percent figure is widely quoted in official NCI documents, its source is elusive and its accuracy is questionable. In her unpublished master's thesis, Lydia Cunningham Rising found support in the medical literature for several different figures, ranging up to 20 percent, although none of the studies she cites is especially persuasive. It is safe to say, however, that only a small minority of adult cancer patients participate in clinical trials.

Chapter 2: *The Structure of Clinical Trials*

1. Two good books on placebos are *The Powerful Placebo: From Ancient Priest to Modern Physician,* by Arthur K. Shapiro and Elaine Shapiro (Baltimore: Johns Hopkins University Press, 1997), and *The Placebo Effect: An Interdisciplinary Exploration,* by Anne Harrington, ed. (Cambridge: Harvard University Press, 1997).

2. Henry K. Beecher, "The Powerful Placebo," *Journal of the American Medical Association* 159 (1955): 1602-06.

3. H. A. Llewellyn-Thomas et al., "Patients' Willingness to Enter Clinical Trials: Measuring the Association with Perceived Benefit and Preference for Decision Participation," *Social Science & Medicine* 32 (1991):35-42.

4. A. B. Benson et al., "Oncologists' Reluctance to Accrue Patients Onto Clinical Trials: An Illinois Cancer Center Study," *Journal of Clinical Oncology* 9 (1991): 2067-75.

5. Benjamin Freedman, "The Ethical Analysis of Clinical Trials: New Lessons For and From Cancer Research," *The Ethics of Research Involving Human Subjects: Facing the 21st Century,* Harold Y. Vanderpool, ed. (Frederick, Maryland: University Publishing Group, Inc., 1996): 319-38.

6. C. Daugherty et al., "Perceptions of Cancer Patients and Their Physicians Involved in Phase I trials," *Journal of Clinical Oncology* 13 (1995): 1062-72.

7. L. H. Yoder et al., "Expectations and Experiences of Patients with Cancer Participating in Phase I Clinical Trials," *Oncology Nursing Forum* 24 (1997): 891-96.

8. This and similar lists of the advantages and disadvantages of different types of clinical trials are adapted in part from Chapter 19 of *Non-Hodgkin's Lymphomas: Making Sense of Diagnosis, Treatment & Options* by Lorraine Johnston (Sebastopol, CA: O'Reilly & Associates, 1999).

9. Lydia Cunningham Rising described Joe's odyssey in personal interviews with the author and in a magazine article (Lydia O. Cunningham, "I Promise I'll Get You Well," *Woman's Day*, October 21, 1986), which she has reprinted on her web site (*http://uhec.udmercy.edu/picct/article1.htm*). A newspaper article describing the science behind and the promise of barrier disruption by focusing on Joe Cunningham's experience in Dr. Edward Neuwelt's clinical trial appeared in the *Los Angeles Times*: Thomas H. Maugh II, "New Tumor Treatment: Breaking the Brain Barrier," *Los Angeles Times*, 21 September 1987.

10. John La Puma, "Physicians' Conflicts of Interest in Post-Marketing Research: What the Public Should Know, and Why Industry Should Tell Them," in Vanderpool, *The Ethics of Research*, 203-19.

11. La Puma, "Physicians' Conflicts of Interest," 203-19.

Chapter 3: *Clinical Trial Ethics*

1. Robert Jay Lifton, *The Nazi Doctors: Medical Killing and the Psychology of Genocide* (New York: Basic Books, 1986).

2. James H. Jones, *Bad Blood: The Tuskegee Syphilis Experiment* (New York: Free Press, 1993).

3. Daniel 1: 12-16 (King James Version).

4. This discussion of the history of clinical trials owes a great deal to David J. Rothman, "Research, Human: Historical Aspects," *Encyclopedia of Bioethics, Revised Edition* (New York: Simon & Schuster Macmillan, 1995): 2248-2258, and Harold Y. Vanderpool, "Introduction and Overview: Ethics, Historical Case Studies, and the Research Enterprise," in Vanderpool, *The Ethics of Research*, 1-30.

5. Rothman, "Research, Human," 2251.

6. Lifton, *The Nazi Doctors*.

7. Albert R. Jonsen, "The Weight and Weighing of Ethical Principles," in Vanderpool, *The Ethics of Research*, 59-82.

8. Rothman, "Research, Human," 2253.

9. Henry K. Beecher, "Ethics and Clinical Research," *New England Journal of Medicine* 274 (1966): 1354-60.

10. Stuart E. Lind, "Financial Issues and Incentives Related to Clinical Research and Innovative Therapies," in Vanderpool, *The Ethics of Research*, 185-202.

11. C. Daugherty et al., "Perceptions of Cancer Patients and Their Physicians Involved in Phase I Trials," *Journal of Clinical Oncology* 13 (1995): 1062-72.

12. Arthur L. Caplan, "Is There a Duty to Serve as a Subject in Biomedical Research?" in Arthur L. Caplan, *If I Were a Rich Man, Could I Buy a Pancreas? and Other Essays on the Ethics of Health Care* (Bloomington, Indiana: University Press, 1992): 85-99.

Chapter 6: *Choosing Possible Trials*

1. "Tough Rules for Kid Drugs," *San Jose Mercury News*, 28 November 1998.

2. Code of Federal Regulations, Title 45, Part 46, Subpart D, Section 46.402, "Federal Policy for the Protection of Human Subjects (Basic Department of Health and Human Services Policy for the Protection of Human Subjects)," Revised June 18, 1991.

3. R. E. Kauffman, "Drug Trials in Children: Ethical, Legal and Practical Issues," *Journal of Clinical Pharmacology* 34 (1994): 296-99.

4. William G. Bartholome, "Ethical Issues in Pediatric Research," in Vanderpool, *The Ethics of Research*, 339-370.

Chapter 7: *Evaluating a Clinical Trial*

1. There's an excellent discussion of this point in Freedman, "The Ethical Analysis of Clinical Trials," 331-35. Freedman refers to several other articles on the consequences of strict exclusion criteria, including K. Antman, et al., "Selection Bias in Clinical Trials," *Journal of Clinical Oncology* 3 (1985): 1142-47; C. B. Begg and P. F. Engstrom, "Eligibility and Extrapolation in Cancer Clinical Trials," *Journal of Clinical Oncology* 5 (1987): 962-68; S. Yusuf et al., "Selection of Patients for Randomized, Controlled Trials: Implications of Wide or Narrow Eligibility Criteria," *Statistics in Medicine* 9 (1990): 73-86; and M. E. Buyse, "The Case For Loose Inclusion Criteria in Clinical Trials," *Acta Chirurgica Belgica* 90, (1990): 129-31.

Chapter 8: *Administration of Clinical Trials*

1. Code of Federal Regulations, Title 45, Part 46, Subpart A, "Federal Policy for the Protection of Human Subjects (Basic Department of Health and Human Services Policy for the Protection of Human Subjects)," Revised June 18, 1991.

2. Charles R. McCarthy, "Challenges to IRBs in the Coming Decades," in Vanderpool, *The Ethics of Research*, 127-44.

3. McCarthy, "Challenges to IRBs," 127-44.

Chapter 9: *Financial Issues*

1. Donald Drake and Marian Uhlman, *Making Medicine, Making Money* (Kansas City, Missouri: Andrews and McMeel, 1993): 5-9.

2. "The Right Prescription," *Fortune*, 21 December 1998, 76.

3. Robert Peer, "Managed-Care Plans Agree to Help Pay the Costs of Their Members in Clinical Trials," *The New York Times*, 9 February 1999.

4. Stuart E. Lind, "Financial Issues and Incentives Related to Clinical Research and Innovative Therapies," in Vanderpool, *The Ethics of Research*, 185-202.

5. This discussion owes a great deal to the excellent chapter on traveling for care in: Lorraine Johnston, *Non-Hodgkin's Lymphomas: Making Sense of Diagnosis, Treatment, and Options* (Sebastopol, CA: O'Reilly & Associates, 1999).

Appendix B: *Critical Public Documents*

1. From "Trials of War Criminals Before the Nuremberg Military Tribunals Under Control Council Law No. 10," Vol. 2, Nuremberg, October 1946 to April 1949. (Washington, DC: US Government Printing Office, 1949): 181-82.

2. Originally published in 44 Federal Register (18 April 1979), 23192-97.

Index

Belmont Report (text of), 42–44, 171–187
Bick, Jane H.
    bringing insurance disputes to media and courts, 150
    negotiating with insurance companies, 147–149
    what insurance should/should not pay for, 145–146
blinding/blinded trials, 18–20

C

cancer center web sites, 66–67
CancerGuide, 18
Caplan, Arthur L.
    duty to serve as research subject if treated at research hospital, 53
Center for Drug Evaluation and Research (FDA), role in approval
    of new therapies, 56, 127–128
CenterWatch, 62, 64–65
children and clinical trials, 93–97
    FDA regulations for, 95
    legal and ethical issues, 95–97
    numbers of participants, 93
    reasons for participation, 93–94
choosing possible clinical trials, 78–80, 91–99
    for children, 93–97
    decision is personal, 8, 97–99
    general considerations in, 92
    options for advanced cancer, 97–99
    See also evaluating clinical trials; special types of trials
clinical research associates, 133
clinical trials, overview of, 1–11
"clinical trials," phrase explained, 2–4
    finding, 6
    participation, lack of, reasons for, ix–xi, 5–7
    participation, reasons for, 7–9
    questions asked and answered, 3
    research and hope for cures, 1–2
    statistics, current, 2
    time needed, 4–5
    traditional vs. alternative medicine, 9–11
Community Clinical Oncology Program (CCOP), 6
complaints about trials, steps in, 54–56
complementary medicine, 11
Consumer Complaint Coordinators (FDA), 56
contract research organizations (CROs), 131–132

Cooperative Oncology Group (COG), 56
costs of trials. See financial issues

D

Data Safety and Monitoring Boards/Data Monitoring Committees,
    139–140
David, Gregory T. and Kuhn, Robert L.
    HMO coverage of lab tests, 146–147
doctors. See physicians
double-blind trials, 19–20
drug companies
    complaining to FDA about, 56
    confidentiality of protocol documents, 119–120
    costs of drug development, 141–142
    limitations on trials, x
    Phase IV studies and marketing, 33–34
    profits of, 143
    testing on children, 94–95
    See also administration of clinical trials; management
        and conduct of trials
Dunn, Steve
    examining protocol document, 117–118
    leaving trials before completion, 18
    Phase II vs. Phases I and III trials, 27

E

eligibility requirements
    examination of, 101–102
    some overly strict, 5, 102–103
email discussion groups on cancer, 69–71
end of treatments, trials possibly appropriate at, 7
ethics of clinical trials
    background and history of trials, 35–44
    Beecher, Henry K., 41–42
    The Belmont Report (text of), 42–44, 171–187
    complaints about trials, steps in, 54–56
    dilemmas for patients, examples of, 50–54
    ethical issues and children in trials, 95–97
        in participant's moving from center to
            center in multicenter trial, 18
        in patients' paying to participate, 155
        in Phase I trials, 21, 22–23

medical devices
    classes of, 87
    trials of, 87–89, 127
Medline, 65–66
multicenter trials, pros and cons of, 138–139

N

National Cancer Institute, 2, 5, 47, 61–64, 132
National Library of Medicine, 65
New Drug Applications (NDAs), 128
news media, 73–75
news release collections, 67–68
Newstracker (Excite), 68–69
Newswise, 68–69
Nuremberg Code (text of), 39–41, 169–171

O

Office for Protection from Research Risks, 55–56
oncologists. See physicians
open-label trials, 18–20
Oster, Nancy
    cancer centers and information about their trials, 67
    changing physicians because of disagreement over
        participation in trials, 60
    medical libraries and research services, 76
overview of clinical trials, 1–11
    "clinical trials," phrase explained, 2–4
    finding, 6
    participation, lack of, reasons for, ix–xi, 5–7
    participation, reasons for, 7–9
    questions asked and answered, 3
    research and hope for cures, 1–2
    statistics, current, 2
    time needed, reasons for, 4–5
    traditional vs. alternative medicine, 9–11

P

participation in clinical trials compensation for, 142–143
    decision is personal, 8, 97–99
    effect of prognosis on, 7, 8–9, 97–99
    lack of, reasons for, ix–xi, 5–7, 102–103
        desire to stop fighting, 7
        difficulty in finding, 6

phases, generally, 13–14
  See also structure of clinical trials
physicians
  consideration of trials urged by, 8–9
  researcher-physicians' conflicts of interest, 44–49
  role in lack of participation in trials, ix–x, 5
  as source of information about trials, 59–61
placebos and placebo effect, 7, 10, 14–16
PPOs. See insurance and insurance providers
PR Newswire, 68–69
prevention and adjuvant trials, 9, 81–84
principal investigator, 133
prognosis, effect of, on participation in clinical trials, 7, 8–9,
  97–99
protocol document, examination of, 116–121
  content of, 116–118
  obstacles to obtaining, 119–121
PubMed, 66

Q

questions before entering trials, 121–125
  for administrators, 123–124
  for doctor and principal investigator, 122–123
  for patient to ask self, 124–125
  tape recording helpful, 121

R

randomization and Phase I trials, 17, 24
  and Phase II trials, 17, 28
  and Phase III trials, 17–18, 30–31, 32
  and phases of trials, overview, 17–18
  in prevention trials, 82
  reluctance toward, 7, 17–18
research services, 76–78
researcher-physicians' conflicts of interest, 44–49
researching clinical trials. See evaluating clinical trials; finding
  clinical trials
Resnik, Ephraim
  adjuvant and prevention trials, 82–84
resources, 161–167
Rising, Lydia Cunningham
  advantages of Phase II trials, 25–26
  importance of honest information about prognosis, 8

importance of patient self-education, 57–58
interacting with researchers, 79–80
risk-taking in choosing trials, 92
role of physicians in finding trials, 59–60

S

Santana, Victor A.
    IRB review of of protocol submissions, 135–136, 139
    issues of children in trials, 93–97
Schine On-Line Services, 77–78
Shoemaker, Dale
    National Cancer Institute "intramural" trials, 132
side effects, fear of, 7
Silvers, Abigail A.
    adjuvant and prevention trials, 82–84
single-blind trials, 19–20
special types of trials, 81–90
    of adjuvant therapies, 9, 81–83
    genetic trials, 89–90
    of medical devices, 87–89, 127
    prevention trials, 82–84
    of supportive therapies, 84–85
    of surgical techniques, 85–86
    See also choosing possible clinical trials; evaluating clinical trials
statistics
    Americans with cancer, number of, 2
    applicants excluded from trials, number of, 102
    cancer survival and death rates, 2
    clinical trials, numbers of, xiii, 91
    clinical trials, success rates, 13–14
    costs of developing new drugs, 141–142
    drug company profits, 143
    drugs as subjects of pediatric trials, number of, 94
    participants in Phase I trials, number of, 21
    participants in Phase II trials, number of, 27
    participants in trials, number of, ix, 5, 93, 189 (note)
    placebos, number responding to, 15
    reasons for entering trials, survey results, 23, 52
    years to bring experimental drug out of lab, number of, 4, 141
structure of clinical trials, 13–34
    blinded and open-label trials, 18–20
    Phase I, 20–25
    Phase II, 25–29

About the Author

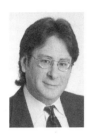

Robert Finn graduated from the University of Chicago with an AB in biological sciences, intending to pursue a career as a research neuroscientist. After several years of graduate studies at the University of California's Department of Psychobiology, he realized he preferred writing to research. Robert left Irvine with an MS degree to pursue a career as a science writer. For a number of years, he worked full-time at the California Institute of Technology in Pasadena writing for Caltech's research magazine, and then for the news media, explaining scientific advances.

Since 1992, Robert has been a full-time freelance writer. His publication credits include articles for *Discover*, *Men's Fitness*, the *Los Angeles Times*, and *The Scientist* (for which he is a contributing editor). Although he has written about many areas of science, he specializes in biomedicine and science policy. He has interviewed close to 1,000 scientists, physicians, and other experts during his career.

Robert has been fascinated with the drug development process and clinical trials since college. Several years ago he worked for a contract research organization, writing chapters for highly technical books intended for scientists interested in clinical trials.

Cancer Clinical Trials: Experimental Treatments & How They Can Help You is Robert's first book. He is now working on a book about organ transplants, which will also be published by O'Reilly.

Colophon

Patient-Centered Guides are about the experience of illness. They contain personal stories as well as a mixture of practical and medical information.

The faces on the covers of our Guides reflect the human side of the information we offer.

The cover of *Cancer Clinical Trials: Experimental Treatments & How They Can Help You,* was designed by Edie Freedman and implemented by Kathleen Wilson, using Adobe Photoshop 5.0 and QuarkXPress 3.32. The cover photo is Copyright © 1994 by Hank Morgan, and is used with permission.

The interior layout of this book was designed by Edie Freedman and implemented by Alicia Cech, using QuarkXPress 3.32. The fonts used are Onyx BT and Berkeley from the Bitstream Foundry.

This book was copyedited by Kristine Simmons and proofread by Sarah Jane Shangraw. Maureen Dempsey, Jane Ellin, and Claire Cloutier LeBlanc conducted quality control checks. Interior composition was done by Alicia Cech. The index was written by Kate Wilkinson.

Patient-Centered Guides™
Questions Answered
Experiences Shared

We are committed to empowering individuals to evolve into informed consumers armed with the latest information and heartfelt support for their journey.

When your life is turned upside down, your need for information is great. You have to make critical medical decisions, often with what seems little to go on. Plus you have to break the news to family, quiet your own fears, cope with symptoms or treatment side effects, figure out how you're going to pay for things, and sometimes still get to work or get dinner on the table.

Patient-Centered Guides provide authoritative information for intelligent information seekers who want to become advocates of their own health. They cover the whole impact of illness on your life. In each book, there's a mix of:

- **Medical background for treatment decisions**
  We can give you information that can help you to intelligently work with your doctor to come to a decision. We start from the viewpoint that modern medicine has much to offer and also discuss complementary treatments. Where there are treatment controversies we present differing points of view.

- **Practical information**
  Once you've decided what to do about your illness, you still have to deal with treatments and changes to your life. We cover day-to-day practicalities, such as those you'd hear from a good nurse or a knowledgeable support group.

- **Emotional support**
  It's normal to have strong reactions to a condition that threatens your life or changes how you live. It's normal that the whole family is affected. We cover issues like the shock of diagnosis, living with uncertainty, and communicating with loved ones.

Each book also contains stories from both patients and doctors — medical "frequent flyers" who share, in their own words, the lessons and strategies they have learned when maneuvering through the often complicated maze of medical information that's available.

We provide information online, including updated listings of the resources that appear in this book. This is freely available for you to print out and copy to share with others, as long as you retain the copyright notice on the printouts.

http://www.patientcenters.com

Other Books in the Series

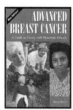

Advanced Breast Cancer
A Guide to Living with Metastatic Disease
By Musa Mayer
ISBN 1-56592-522-X, Paperback 6" x 9", 542 pages,
$19.95

"An excellent book...if knowledge is power, this book will be good medicine."

—David Spiegel, MD
Stanford University
Author,
Living Beyond Limits

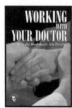

Working with Your Doctor
Getting the Healthcare You Deserve
By Nancy Keene
ISBN 1-56592-273-5, Paperback, 6" x 9", 382 pages,
$15.95

"Working with Your Doctor fills a genuine need for patients and their family members caught up in this new and intimidating age of impersonal, economically-driven health care delivery."

—James Dougherty, MD
Emeritus Professor of Surgery,
Albany Medical College

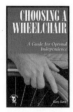

Choosing a Wheelchair
A Guide for Optimal Independence
By Gary Karp
ISBN 1-56592-411-8, Paperback, 5" x 8", 192 pages,
$9.95

"I love the idea of putting knowledge often possessed only by professionals into the hands of new consumers. Gary Karp has done it. This book will empower people with disabilities to make informed equipment choices."

—Barry Corbet
Editor,
New Mobility Magazine

Patient-Centered Guides
Published by O'Reilly & Associates, Inc.
Our products are available at a bookstore near you.
For information: **800-998-9938** • **707-829-0515** • **info@oreilly.com**
101 Morris Street • Sebastopol • CA • 95472-9902

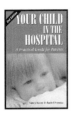

Your Child in the Hospital
A Practical Guide for Parents, Second Edition
By Nancy Keene and Rachel Prentice
ISBN 1-56592-573-4, Paperback, 5" x 8", 176 pages,
$11.95

"When your child is ill or injured, the hospital setting can be overwhelming. Here is a terrific 'road map' to help keep families 'on track.'"

—James B. Fahner, MD
Division Chief,
Pediatric Hematology/Oncology,
DeVos Children's Hospital,
Grand Rapids, Michigan

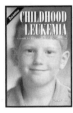

Childhood Leukemia
A Guide for Families, Friends, and Caregiver, 2nd Edition
By Nancy Keene
ISBN 1-56592-632-3, Paperback, 6" x 9", 564 pages,
$24.95

"What's so compelling about Childhood Leukemia is the amount of useful medical information and practical advice it contains. Keene avoids jargon and lays out what's needed to deal with the medical system."

—The Washington Post

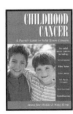

Childhood Cancer
A Parent's Guide to Solid Tumor Cancers
By Nancy Keene
ISBN 1-56592-531-9, Paperback, 6" x 9", 540 pages,
$24.95

"I recommend [this book] most highly for those in need of high level, helpful knowledge that will empower and help parents and caregivers to cope."

—Mark Greenberg, MD
Professor of Pediatrics,
University of Toronto

Patient-Centered Guides
Published by O'Reilly & Associates, Inc.
Our products are available at a bookstore near you.
For information: 800-998-9938 • 707-829-0515 • info@oreilly.com
101 Morris Street • Sebastopol • CA • 95472-9902

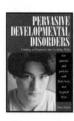

Pervasive Developmental Disorders
Finding a Diagnosis and Getting Help
By Mitzi Waltz
ISBN 1-56592-530-0, Paperback, 6" x 9", 592 pages,
$24.95

"Mitzi Waltz's book provides clear, informative, and comprehensive information on every relevant aspect of PDD. Her in-depth discussion will help parents and professionals develop a clear understanding of the issues and, consequently, they will be able to make informed decisions about various interventions. A job well done!"

—Dr. Stephen M. Edelson
Director,
Center for the Study of Autism,
Salem, Oregon

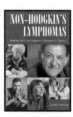

Non-Hodgkin's Lymphomas
Making Sense of Diagnosis, Treatment & Options
By Lorraine Johnston
ISBN 1-56592-444-4, Paperback, 6" x 9", 584 pages,
$24.95

"When I gave this book to one of our patients, there was an instant, electric connection. A sense of enlightenment came over her while she absorbed the information. It was thrilling to see her so sparked with new energy and focus."

—Susan Weisberg, LCSW
Clinical Social Worker,
Stanford University Medical Center

Patient-Centered Guides
Published by O'Reilly & Associates, Inc.
Our products are available at a bookstore near you.
For information: **800-998-9938** • **707-829-0515** • **info@oreilly.com**
101 Morris Street • Sebastopol • CA • 95472-9902

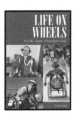

Life on Wheels
For the Active Wheelchair User
By Gary Karp
ISBN 1-56592-253-0, Paperback, 6" x 9", 576 pages,
$24.95

*"I think a book like this should be given to everyone in the
rehab hospital ... it offers the broadest perspective of life on
wheels that I've ever seen."*

—Michelle Gittler, MD
Director,
Resident Training Program,
Schwab Rehab Hospital

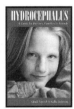

Hydrocephalus
A Guide for Patients, Families & Friends
By Chuck Toporek and Kellie Robinson
ISBN 1-56592-410-X, Paperback, 6" x 9", 384 pages,
$19.95

*"Toporek, a medical editor, and wife Robinson, a writer and
hydrocephalus patient, fill a void of information on
hydrocephalus (water on the brain) for the lay reader. Highly
recommended for public and academic libraries."*

—Library Journal

*"In this book, the authors have provided a wonderful entry into
the world of hydrocephalus to begin to remedy the neglect of
this important condition. We are immensely grateful to them
for their groundbreaking effort."*

—Peter M. Black, MD, PhD
Franc D. Ingraham Professor of Neurosurgery,
Harvard Medical School
Neurosurgeon-in-Chief,
Brigham and Women's Hospital,
Children's Hospital,
Boston, Massachusetts

Patient-Centered Guides

Published by O'Reilly & Associates, Inc.
Our products are available at a bookstore near you.
For information: **800-998-9938 • 707-829-0515 • info@oreilly.com**
101 Morris Street • Sebastopol • CA • 95472-9902

We Care About What You Think

Which book did this card come from?

_____

Why did you purchase this book?
- ☐ I am directly impacted
- ☐ A family member or friend is directly impacted
- ☐ I am a health-care practitioner looking for information to recommend to patients and their families
- ☐ Other _____

How did you first find out about the book?
- ☐ Recommended by a friend/colleague/family member
- ☐ Recommended by a doctor/nurse
- ☐ Saw it in a bookstore
- ☐ Online
- ☐ Other _____

- ☐ *Please send me the Patient-Centered Guides catalog.*

What sources do you use to gather your medical information?
- ☐ Friends/family   ☐ A library
- ☐ Your doctor   ☐ Your nurse(s)
- ☐ Television (which shows?) _____
- ☐ Newspapers (which newspapers?) _____
- ☐ Magazines (which magazines?) _____
- ☐ Newsletters (which newsletters) _____
- ☐ The Internet (which newsgroups, mailing lists or Web sites?) _____
- ☐ Support Groups (which groups?) _____
- ☐ Other _____

What other medical conditions are of concern to you, your family, and community?

_____

_____

Name _____ Company/Organization (Optional) _____

Address _____

City _____ State _____ Zip/Postal Code _____ Country _____

Telephone _____ Internet or other email address (specify network) _____

Ten Patient Rights

1. Receive considerate and respectful care.

2. Obtain complete information on illness and treatment.

3. Participate in treatment decisions.

4. Give informed consent.

5. Refuse any treatment.

6. Receive reasonable medical care and skill.

7. Wait only a reasonable amount of time.

8. Have your records kept confidential.

9. Get copies of requested records.

10. Have an advocate with you.

Patient-Centered Guides
800-998-9938

BUSINESS REPLY MAIL

FIRST CLASS MAIL   PERMIT NO. 80   SEBASTOPOL, CA

Postage will be paid by addressee

O'Reilly & Associates, Inc.

101 Morris Street

Sebastopol, CA 95472-9902

Attn: Patient-Centered Guides